FINDING STRENGTH
A Mother and Daughter's Story of Childhood Cancer

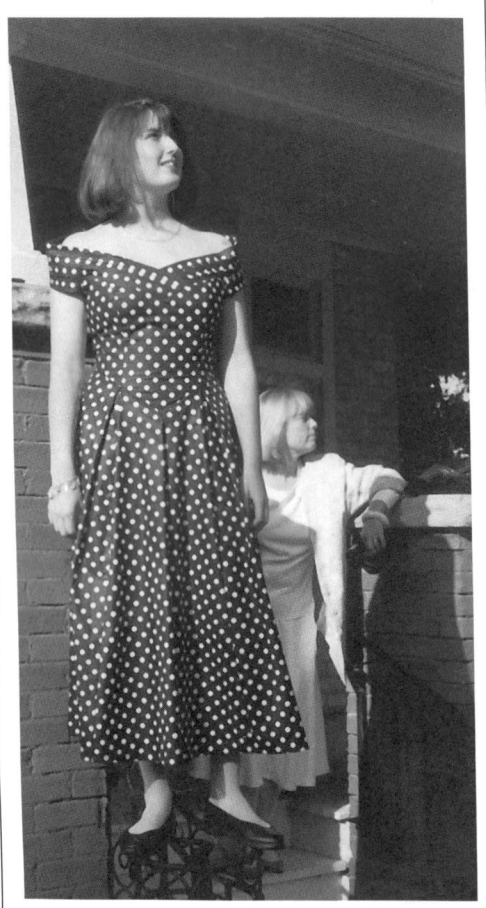

Lauren and Juanne on the front porch at home on the evening of Lauren's grade eight graduation.

FINDING STRENGTH
A Mother and Daughter's Story of Childhood Cancer

Juanne Nancarrow Clarke
with Lauren Nancarrow Clarke

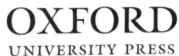

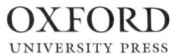

70 Wynford Drive, Don Mills, Ontario M3C 1J9
www.oupcan.com

Oxford University Press is a department of the University of Oxford.
It furthers the University's objective of excellence in research, scholarship,
and education by publishing worldwide in

Oxford New York

Athens Auckland Bangkok Bogotá Buenos Aires Calcutta
Cape Town Chennai Dar es Salaam Delhi Florence Hong Kong Istanbul
Karachi Kuala Lumpur Madrid Melbourne Mexico City Mumbai
Nairobi Paris São Paulo Singapore Taipei Tokyo Toronto Warsaw

with associated companies in Berlin Ibadan

Oxford is a trade mark of Oxford University Press
in the UK and in certain other countries

Published in Canada
by Oxford University Press

Copyright © Oxford University Press Canada 1999

The moral rights of the author have been asserted

Database right Oxford University Press (maker)

First published 1999

All rights reserved. No part of this publication may be reproduced,
stored in a retrieval system, or transmitted, in any form or by any means,
without the prior permission in writing of Oxford University Press,
or as expressly permitted by law, or under terms agreed with the appropriate
reprographics rights organization. Enquiries concerning reproduction
outside the scope of the above should be sent to the Rights Department,
Oxford University Press, at the address above.

You must not circulate this book in any other binding or cover
and you must impose this same condition on any acquirer.

Canadian Cataloguing in Publication Data

Clarke, Juanne N. (Juanne Nancarrow), 1944-
Finding strength : a mother and daughter's story of childhood cancer
Includes bibliographical references.
ISBN 0-19-541482-9
1. Clarke, Lauren Nancarrow - Health. 2. Leukemia in children - Patients -
Canada - Biography. I. Clarke, Lauren Nancarrow. II. Title
RJ416.L4C527 1999   362.1'989299419'0092   C99-931725-3

Cover & Text Design: Brett Miller
Cover photo by: Marion Campbell, Lauren's stepmother, 'extraordinaire'

1 2 3 4 - 02 01 00 99
This book is printed on permanent (acid-free) paper ∞
Printed in Canada

Contents

Preface, vii

Acknowledgements, ix

1. Spinach and Raisins for Lunch, 1
2. Choreographing and Telling the Diagnosis, 16
3. Acknowledging the Diagnosis, Telling Others, and Thinking about Causation, 31
4. Remission Induction: Boot Camp in Hospital Living, 46
5. Mistakes Are Routine: Confusion, Contradiction, and the Unpredictable Cycle, 73
6. Clinic Visits: Here or There?, 91
7. Back to Normal?, 108
8. Committing Complementary Care, 124
9. How Has Cancer Changed Your Life?, 139
10. Treatment Ends?, 151
11. Cancer Charities for Kids: Answers to Dreams and Wishes?, 160
12. Looking Back and Looking Forward, 181

Lauren's Epilogue, 192

Bibliography, 203

Appendix: Resources for Childhood Cancer, 210

Preface

This book started out as notes to myself. I started keeping notes as a way of remembering and as a way of coping with some of the things that were happening. Writing seemed to give me some sense of distance and control. The personal story soon turned to questions. I wanted to know why certain things were happening as they were. Why did we not know that my daughter Lauren was sick for such a long time? Why did we sit where we sat, ritualistically, when given the diagnosis? What was known about the causes of leukemia? How common was the disease? Was its incidence increasing? Why did I see a mouse on the floor of the pediatric oncology ward? Why did nurses come to work sick? Why were a few doctors so difficult and others so wonderful, and why did their interpersonal style seem to matter so much? Why was it difficult to get information on the childhood cancer charities? These are a few of the questions that I became intrigued with as I wrote out my experiences with Lauren's diagnosis with leukemia.

From the vantage point of a mother of a child with leukemia I found that I was quite critical of a number of previously taken-for-granted realities. I take issue with the focus and the findings of some of the research literature in my own field of medical sociology, as well as in the psychology literature. I find myself frustrated with the continuing focus in epidemiological literature on a wide range of potential carcinogens in the absence of either conclusive findings or policy advocacy. There is clearly enough known about a large number of carcinogens to ban their presence in the food we eat, the land on which we live, the water we drink and in which we swim, and the air we breathe. Likewise, I am amazed at the size of the charities industry in Canada and its relative freedom from regulation. I am dismayed by the effects of the cutbacks to the health-care system, especially as these impact on the well-being of the most vulnerable members of our society.

In sum, what began as notes to myself became a quest for answers to some difficult questions. At the same time, Lauren had been doing her own searching and writing. She created a magazine for children with cancer as a project for a creative writing course in her final year of high school, a time that coincided with the initial diagnosis and first year of treatment; she continued to write poetry; and later she wrote several articles on 'living with cancer' for her university newspaper. Some of this material is included here to lend another perspective to my own point of view as a mother and a sociologist. In addition, Lauren read drafts of the manuscript and has added footnotes to offer yet more of a daughter's and patient's perspective. We hope our story will shed light on any such journey you must make.

Acknowledgements

Before I acknowledge those who helped specifically with this book, I want to thank all of the doctors and nurses we met over the course of diagnosis and treatment of Lauren's leukemia. My admiration and respect for the work they do has grown immeasurably over the past few years. I did not know personally and I had not thought much about the enormous commitment required by health-care professionals. The nurses and doctors we met had dedicated their lives, and not just their hours at work, to their professions. They often worked long hours, long after many of us would normally be at home sleeping, taking care of these very vulnerable children. They often worked in situations of crisis, and had to respond to solve sudden problems quickly. They did this in the awful context of a decline in government support for their work, of cutbacks in service, in beds, in personnel. Nurses, who just a few years earlier worked in the security of a full-time position with essential benefits continuing indefinitely, were facing the possibility of lay-offs. This was at a time when the hospital sector was contracting as precipitously as a balloon once untied. Nurses were being let go. Sometimes they were later hired back on a part-time basis, without benefits and at a lower wage. Most new graduates could hope only for part-time work without benefits. Those who kept their jobs or came back to the hospital worked with fewer and fewer staff. It was not unheard of for a nurse on night duty to spend the night running from patient to patient without time to stop for a break or to make the growing numbers of notes required.

The doctors, too, suffered from the cutbacks in the hospitals. In the clinic at the hospital where Lauren was diagnosed the number of physicians on staff had more than halved in the previous decade, as had the number of support staff. Yet, these doctors were expected, because they were associated with a university hospital, not only to care for critically and sometimes terminally ill children (and their distraught parents, step-parents, siblings, etc.) day and night, but also to do research, to teach, and to 'publish or perish'. The doctors also worked in a society that seemed increasingly to value them less as an organized group. They were on the defensive. They had lost a province-wide strike in the mid-1980s because of the lack of public support for their strike position. They spoke out against the government cutbacks, but the health economists and administrators seem to have more influence.

Not only were there fewer nursing, medical, and other staff, but the physical facilities were sometimes inadequate. At times there were no beds in the system for a child with cancer and a fever, who needed to be hospitalized in order to receive intravenous antibiotics to prevent the spread of a potentially life-threatening infection. These were hard times in the Ontario system for the doctors and nurses, who gave so much and continued to do so under extreme stress. Work in oncology, particularly with children, is already among the most stressful of medical and nursing work. When you add the dire threats to the hospital system within which they work and the widespread decrease in public trust, it is more than understandable that we as patients and family suffered not only from the disease and the physical effects of the treatments but from the outrageous and violent changing of the hospital system, sometimes via the expressed interpersonal stress of doctors and nurses.

At times I am quite critical of the experiences that we had at the hands of the medical personnel. This part of the story needs to be told. It did happen. But there were many, many more positive experiences of interaction with the medical personnel. When all is said and done, we are grateful to everyone with whom we had an encounter. We believe that they were all doing their best, that they were in this work fundamentally to help sick and suffering people.

Lauren received most of her treatment on an out-patient basis at the local hospital. Words cannot express our gratitude to Patti Banbury, Brenda Rice, Linda Szozda, and Dr Ian Wilson.

Mary Murray, our home-care co-ordinator, was a constant source of encouragement to me over that first eight months or so when Lauren periodically had a nurse come by to inject a particular medication. After practising first on an orange, Lauren later learned to inject herself. But in the meantime, many was the morning when I called Mary to ask if she could order the pump, which we picked up at the local hospital to take down to the big city hospital, that I talked and talked while Lauren slept upstairs. Mary had lots of experience with this disease and its treatments. She was another person upon whom I relied.

I also want to thank family, friends, and colleagues too numerous to mention for all of the kindnesses shown to us as we passed through this time. A number of the teachers from Lauren's high school, especially Pierre Sandor, Jim Weber, and Don Woodley, seemed to care for Lauren as if she were one of their own children.

Several people have helped specifically in the writing of the book. Leslie Morgenson has been involved from the beginning collecting research articles, calling charities, and contacting pediatric oncology organizations. Leslie put together most of the section on resources. Leslie, along with Sue Bodell, Jo Levy Sack, and Frances Humphries, read parts of the manuscript and offered ideas, support, and encouragement.

Richard Tallman, the editor for Oxford, read the book as a parent as well as an editor and helped me to clarify ideas and to read what I had written as a reader might. Laura Macleod from Oxford read the first few chapters and responded enthusiastically, asking that her colleagues read the manuscript. Phyllis Wilson, on Laura's recommendation, read the same chapters and agreed to its publication.

I am always grateful to be working at Wilfrid Laurier University. It has been and continues to be a wonderful place to teach and do research. I find the balance between teaching and research stimulating and challenging. I would like to thank my department colleagues and students as well as the administrators of the university for allowing me the time I needed to take care of Lauren.

Finally, Lauren and I would like to thank you, the reader, for taking time to read our story.

Juanne Nancarrow Clarke
April 1999

Dear Reader,

Thank-you for opening these pages and reading this book. I am privileged that you took time to hear my mom's and my story. This is not an 'it could happen to you' tale or a story about 'how not to get cancer'. Rather, it is an exploration of a time in our lives when most of our control was taken away from us and we simply survived. It is a book about what was good and what went wrong in my medical treatment. It tells the story of one specific incident that extends out to many other larger implications. This book is a testimony to the fact that life goes on, that we can recover, and that there is grace.

The structure of the book follows the pattern of my mom's primary writing and investigation on health. Along the way I have added thoughts, contradictions, and my emotions to my mom's work. I have written an epilogue to this book.

Please find strength in these words that my mom and I have written. They are written both for you and for us.

Lauren Nancarrow Clarke
April 1999

Chapter 1

Spinach and Raisins for Lunch

It was the summer of 1995. My 17-year-old daughter and I were spending this time in the city together. Lauren wanted to get a lot of sunshine, relaxation, and exercise. She was working at a French camp during the day, about three miles from home. An easy bike ride, or so we thought. Lauren intended to ride back and forth to camp for the three weeks. I was planning to ride with her, just for the exercise.

On the Sunday before the camp was to begin, we found its location by driving our car through the quiet, still, and sunny suburban streets where the camp was to be held at a public school and in its playground. We worked out a route and were prepared to start early to ride the next morning to make sure we were there by 8:30 with plenty of time to spare. But the next morning dawned grey and rainy, and so I drove Lauren to camp. The following day, again, it was raining, and the next. And so by Thursday we were planning to bike, but Lauren said she was tired and would prefer to drive and walk part of the way. We finally left home too late to walk at all and I drove her to the front of the school. As it turned out, the furthest Lauren ever walked to camp that summer was one block.

One day we set out to ride our bikes, a 10-minute ride, over to the grocery and video store. Lauren was exhausted on our way home. She had to stop and sit on the ground for a while to recoup. Still, the last thing I thought of was that she was sick or even 'really' sick. Instead, this tiredness led me to make efforts to help her build herself up. We were so used to thinking about and acting on prevention and health promotion suggestions that the idea of sickness did not occur to either of us. More vitamins, iron, rest, exercise, fun, good food: these were the remedies to which we turned.

At the time, I was a wee bit concerned about her health but I saw the problem as definitely fixable. She had never been terribly active, by 'nature' or inclination. I still ruminate about how long she may have had leukemia before we knew. Retrospectively, there were lots of signs, but at the time they seemed normal or only a little off normal, but there was no inkling to me—ever—that she had something seriously wrong.[1] Leukemia did not enter even the furthest reaches of my awareness.

The French day camp was the first three weeks of July. Her tiredness continued after the camp. I continued to try to encourage her to relax, eat well, and exercise. She began to work out at home on the exercise bike and to walk regularly. Her goal was an hour of exercise of one sort or another each day, and she continued all summer to exercise about one hour daily. My concerns about her health remained, but I was not medically oriented yet—just preoccupied about her well-being and getting her to feel better and more energetic.

Her best friend, Meaghan, had left for Thailand for a year in June and her boyfriend, Michael, had gone out West to a summer science 'intensive' for the month of July. I remember interpreting some of her lack of energy to underlying feelings of loss associated with the departures of her two closest friends. In August, she went away for a week to a cottage in Muskoka with her dad and stepmother, Marian. I recall feeling relieved when she reported that she had felt well at Marian's cottage and had walked for at least an hour a day.[2] Whew! The next week, Jess (Lauren's sister, who is four years older), who had finished her summer job as a camp counsellor, Lauren, and I went to our cottage.

One day Jess wanted to go for a hike and so we drove to a park with rapids, and falls, and a wide and energetic river. We played in the

---

[1] My own feelings parallel those of my mom in this regard. I was (and am once again) a vegetarian, and so I thought that perhaps I wasn't getting the proper nutrients. I was busy and so I thought I had reason to be tired. No one in my immediate family had ever been truly sick, and therefore there was no reason to suspect that I was.

[2] During these walks, out on the highway, in the bright sun, I would run a longer and longer distance each day. At the end of these runs my face was always beet red. This seemed normal for my exertion level. What wasn't normal was how white my skin was under the red. It was so white, in fact, that Marian was concerned.

water for a bit, then Jess and I went hiking. Lauren was exhausted—she lay on a blanket on a hill, reading and resting. Jess and I, aware of Lauren's tiredness, were gone only about an hour. Afterwards we went to a lakeside town for fresh fish and chips. Lauren was so tired we had to drive right down to the dock—usually we parked in the small downtown area and walked the quarter of a mile or so to the 'fish shack'. But still I wasn't about to really worry.

Suddenly, it was September and school started. Jess went back to university, and Lauren again began her busyness with the 7:15 meetings and early school starting time. She was on student council and in a number of clubs and often had to be at school very early. I drove her and so I got up when she did. She continued to feel tired and we explained it as the early start to the day (but then, I wasn't tired).

Lauren organized the 'AIDS walk' for her school early in October and about 20 of her schoolmates went over to the nearby park to compete against other schools in seeing who was able to get the largest number of participants out to raise money by walking 10 kilometres for AIDS. The organizers had balloons and bands to welcome the walkers. Each school team warmed up together. I remember Lauren actively leading the wild, exuberant warm-up with her teammates. A bit later we all set off on the walk. Lauren and her team were walking ahead of us. My friend and I were pulling up behind. But when we reached the first refreshment stop, just 15 minutes or so from where we all began, Lauren was sitting on the grass, her boyfriend, Michael, beside her. My friend and I stopped. Lauren said she was exhausted. She was dizzy and seeing spots. Michael said that he was going to leave her there and get his car to take her home. She had decided that she had better rest for the afternoon and I said I'd walk for her the rest of the way.

School went on for one more week and Lauren did, too. She reported feeling tired and having to stop on the way up the stairs in the old, many-storeyed school, but she carried on. One day she had a swollen gland in her neck and she was worried. I took her to a doctor at the local urgent-care clinic, who said 'it looks like a virus'. Another day a teacher told her she looked 'green'. Finally, about five weeks after school started—on Thanksgiving weekend during dinner preparations—I told my sister, Cindy, and my mother, both of whom were nurses, that Lauren was tired. My mother looked under her eyes and found that the skin under her eyelids was very pale.

My sister suggested that we go to the doctor to see if she was anemic. She had been taking some iron supplements but Cindy said that sometimes teenage girls needed much larger, therapeutic, doses of iron. I was planning to make an appointment with our doctor sometime that week. On the Tuesday morning, after Thanksgiving Monday, Lauren had to sit down in the middle of her morning shower.[3] Her head felt dizzy and she just wasn't well. I was going to take her to school and meanwhile call the doctor and be available to pick her up for the appointment, if he could fit her in and if she continued to feel sick.[4] She tried to get dressed but was too tired, and so we decided that we had better not wait for an appointment.

We went immediately to the urgent-care clinic—but we didn't have Lauren's health card. There was a little bit of commotion until she remembered that her health-card number should be there from previous visits. We not only had been there a few weeks earlier when Lauren had had a swollen gland, but she had been there in early June with a fever and bronchitis. She had cleaned out a cupboard at her high school—one that had not been cleaned for many years—and had reacted violently to the dust, dirt, and whatever else was in the cupboard. Cleaning the cupboard occurred on a Friday. By Saturday she was so sick that her dad and Marian had taken her to this clinic where she was prescribed an antibiotic. I remember wondering at the time whether or not she had needed this drug. I was very concerned about their tendency to be overused and mis-

---

3 Who has ever heard of a healthy 17-year-old needing to sit down in the middle of a shower? And this Tuesday morning was not the first occasion. I had been sitting down in the shower periodically from the spring of that year. It, along with many other abnormalities, became routine. Shampoo, sit down, rinse, condition, sit down . . . .

4 This may seem odd—that I would be planning on going to school when I appeared to be so sick—but I never wanted to miss school, especially if there was some extracurricular activity that I was participating in or leading. Normally, I would have insisted on going to school . . . but not that day.

used. I thought that patients were too ready to ask for antibiotics and physicians were too ready to give them out. I was worried about the long-term effects of taking too many antibiotics when they weren't absolutely indicated as a result of tests to determine the type of bacteria in an infection. I was concerned about their ultimate effectiveness—when and if they were ever really needed. But I wasn't concerned that Lauren was 'really' sick, although, come to think of it, she never really recovered from this illness episode.

Even today, as I write this another new study is being reported in the local press about the dangers of excess antibiotic usage. In this case, the research published in the prestigious *Journal of the American Medical Association,* conducted by a team of Canadian researchers at the University of Ottawa and the University of Manitoba, reports that the current 10-day course of antibiotics for typical ear infections can be cut down to five days. As ear infections in children are a major cause of antibiotic use (this article reports that 60 to 80 per cent of children will have ear infections before the age of seven), cutting the length of treatment for just this one medical problem could have a significant impact on the overall rate of prescriptions of antibiotics (Bueckert, 1998: 8).

The doctor on duty at the urgent-care clinic asked what was

It Can Happen To Anyone—It Happened To Me

... In the spring of 1995 ... I developed a bronchial infection and was sick for two weeks. My doctor prescribed some easy, quick-acting antibiotics to cure me.... What followed ... were three months of me feeling more tired than usual. Nothing happened that, in and of itself, would cause alarm, but eventually things built up to reveal a larger problem.

I was a French camp counsellor that summer. We did a lot of different activities: singing in French, making slime out of corn starch and water, playing soccer, and other things of that nature. I found that after the first five minutes or so of chasing children I was exhausted. I blamed it on the sun, not having eaten enough breakfast, anything that could have been true once or twice, but not repeatedly. What ended up happening was that my partner would take the outdoor activities as primary counsellor and I would do the indoor. This eliminated the 'problem', or so I thought.

Later that same summer I went on a hike with my family. My 'hike' consisted of finding the start of the trail, looking at the map, and deciding that I was too tired to walk it. I ended up sitting, in the shade, for the hour and a half that the rest of my family walked. Even when they came back, my stroll over to the concession stand to get a pop for my sister was exhausting. This was definitely not the way a healthy 17-year-old was supposed to be feeling.

Continually, throughout this period, I needed to sit down while taking showers. After about three minutes I would need to turn off the water and sit until I felt strong enough to stand up and rinse off. Again, this was not normal, but at the time I made excuses.

Summer ended, and I went back to school. There, I needed to rest after climbing from my first-floor English class to my locker on the second floor. There, I was told by a science teacher in front of the class that I looked green. I shrugged this off, thinking that the teacher was impolite, but not incorrect. Later that week a different teacher said that I looked pale. I was (and am again) a vegetarian, so I thought that my paleness was due to anemia, caused by my diet.

Eventually, I noticed an enlarged lymph node on my neck. My mom and I went to a walk-in clinic. We were quickly and efficiently (as those clinics are) dealt with and sent forth as healthy into the healthy world. The doctor told us to come back if it didn't go away on its own. It went away in a few days.

Three weeks later, after further incidents of flashing lights and perpetually needing to sit down to clear my head, I woke up thinking that something was wrong. Placed together like this on a page it is so blatant, so apparent that my conclusion was correct.

However, during that time, everything could be (and was) explained away. The flu, my vegetarianism, waking up too early and staying too late at school: all of this could add up to what was happening to me on a daily basis. But not for three months. I decided that I couldn't go to school that day. This was after attempting to shower, and needing to sit down as soon as I put the water on, after about five seconds.

> My mom decided to take me back to the walk-in clinic (we were in between doctors at the time, ours being newly retired)....
>
> Less than three hours after I had gone in to get my blood taken, the doctor was calling. This seemed a little strange. Now, I am so thankful for that doctor's action; he helped get the ball rolling for my (future) cure. My mom answered the phone and the doctor said: 'I think there might be something serious here.'
>
> As we know, he was quite right.
>
> From *Imprint* (University of Waterloo), 10 Oct. 1997.

wrong with Lauren and she and I explained that she was 'really' tired all the time and pale. I said that I wanted him to order a blood test in case she was anemic. He said to me, 'But you're pale, too', and I said, 'Yes, but I have lots of energy and endurance.' Then he said, 'Oh, okay'—and ordered a blood test.[5] We went home, Lauren lay down on the couch to read, and I sat at my desk doing some work. Within an hour the doctor called and said he had the results of the blood test. 'I think it's serious', he said, 'a problem with her bone marrow.' I asked what he meant, what could it be, what sort of problem he was talking about. 'Leukemia or aplastic anemia,' he answered. My stomach dropped and I swallowed deeply—tears came to my eyes—but I didn't really believe it. The doctor said he would make an appointment with a hemotologist for as soon as possible and would call back to let us know when it would be. Within a couple of hours he called back. Lauren had an appointment for a bone marrow aspiration for 9:30 the next morning. I was in shock but still didn't believe it. He was overreacting, I told myself. He was looking for the worst. So I made Lauren a bowl of spinach for lunch with a bunch of raisins for dessert. It was anemia, these foods were supposed to be iron-rich, and we were going to get serious about treating it.

---

5   I did not have the energy during this test to keep my head off my elbow on the desk. Here I sat in a public office too tired to keep up the appearance of being well. Something was gravely wrong.

The afternoon passed. I eventually told Lauren what the doctor had said and that he had set up an appointment for a bone marrow aspiration for the next day.[6] I still really did not think that 'it' was happening. I continued to work at my desk. Lauren lay on the couch watching television and then, when school was out, talking on the phone to her friends. I called Lauren's French teacher to say that she was going to be unable to make a presentation in school the next day. I had agreed to be interviewed by the editor of a local health magazine; but I had forgotten. She came to the door. I still didn't believe the as yet indeterminate news. Lauren was watching late afternoon TV and talking on the phone, so I went through with the interview. My only serious concern was that the person doing the interview had a cold sore. I didn't want to get it from her and pass it on to Lauren when her health already seemed compromised.

It took about six hours for me to admit to myself that the bone marrow aspiration was real and that they were really looking for leukemia or another serious disease.[7] Then I called my sister in a nearby city for advice—her friend, 'Suzi', across the street, was a pediatric oncologist and worked as a researcher rather than a practitioner at the university hospital. I had gone over to the clinic to get the blood counts earlier so that I could take these to the local doctor who was scheduled to do the bone marrow aspiration the next day. My sister called her neighbour, Suzi, to explain what had happened. She asked about Lauren's blood results. I opened the envelope and read the numbers to my sister, who later passed them on to Suzi. I had no idea what they meant. Suzi said she would arrange to have Lauren seen at a big city hospital, which had a pedi-

---

6 That's not how I remember it. When the doctor called Mom was helping me write out my résumé for applying for first-year university scholarships. She was typing what I was dictating because I was too weak to sit up and do it myself. I was lying at her feet and I could hear her voice and see her tears appear. I asked her what was wrong and she told me immediately. We went to our living room and hugged on the couch, crying for a few minutes. Then we resolved that the doctor was wrong—I was only anemic. We would take care of the problem ourselves—hence the lunch.

7 I never thought it could be something serious until the doctor told me that I had leukemia. For me, serious illness was just not a possibility. I had a life to live, things to do, work for school that needed to be finished. I could not possibly be really sick.

atric-oncology unit, the next day. She reassured me by saying that if it were her child, she'd go there. She also reiterated what the physician had said earlier on the phone—if Lauren's temperature were to go above 38.5 degrees Celsius we were to go immediately to the big city hospital and she would arrange that we be admitted.

Lauren's boyfriend, Michael, was in the family room with her at this time. I told them about the news. I had purchased a thermometer earlier in the day when the urgent-care physician had made the same point—to go to the hospital if she got a fever. Lauren and Michael took her temperature because she felt hot. It was 38.6. I called my sister and her neighbour said she would make arrangements for Lauren to be admitted that evening. Still in shock, we collected a pillow and blanket for the car, some toiletries, and a change of clothes for each of us. With Michael's help, we packed up the car, rolled back the front seat, and made Lauren as comfortable as possible. I promised I'd stay with her in the hospital and down we went to be admitted. Neither of us was really worried. We were sure it must be a mistake but we headed off—not just in case, but in any case.

Why did it take us so long to take Lauren's symptoms seriously? Was I negligent? Was Lauren denying? Were we acting unusually foolishly in the face of what turned out to be a serious, life-threatening illness? Sociologists and health psychologists have found that most people tend to normalize vague symptoms as long as possible. The symptoms tend to be thought of as temporary, or not so bad or controllable with will and a close attention to health-promoting behaviours. Lauren's major symptom was tiredness. Who has not felt tired? Who has not felt an ongoing fatigue or ennui and rationalized it to be the result of an unusually busy or stressful time? Even when a symptom or a series of symptoms begins more dramatically and more precipitously, people tend to justify and rationalize the symptoms as temporary or perhaps normal 'for my age, my current level of stress', for instance. This general theory tends also to be true of as serious a disease as cancer and, particularly because it is so infrequent, of childhood cancer. Research on childhood cancer and its onset is consistent. In most cases the young person experiences a series of seemingly mild, vague symptoms for a time before being taken to the doctor. The most common symptoms of leukemia are tiredness, fevers, easy bruising and bleeding, bone pain, enlarged lymph nodes, and swollen glands. Each of these alone is, at times, normal or indicative of mild and self-limiting illnesses. Which of us has never had these ordinary symptoms?

Nancy Keene (1997: 1) describes the difficulties of diagnosis:

> Diagnosis of leukemia is extremely difficult because many symptoms mimic those of normal childhood illnesses. The onset of the disease can be slow and insidious or very rapid. Initially, children begin to tire easily. And rest often. Frequently, they have a fever which comes and goes. Interest in eating gradually diminishes, but only some people lose weight. Parents usually notice pale skin and occasional bruising. Some children develop back, leg and joint pain which makes it difficult for them to walk. Often lymph nodes in the neck and groin become enlarged, and the upper abdomen protrudes due to enlargement of the spleen and liver. Children become cranky and irritable, and occasional nose bleeds develop.

In our case, unlike many others, the only 'symptoms' we were aware of were tiredness and palour. Still, that first doctor took me, the parent, seriously and ordered a blood test when it was requested of him. He was reluctant. He did not know us and did not know if Lauren and I were frequent doctor shoppers. He could not see anything unusual. Being tired could easily have been viewed as a psychosomatic symptom. But this doctor listened and took the requested action. Then, as soon as he had received the blood counts, he acted promptly and responsibly.[8]

The fact that there was one easily accomplished test—the

---

8   I want to call him a hero. I want to thank him again and again for his outstanding work—yet, really, this is not justified. As a doctor he should have done what he did. As a doctor he did his job. The fact that I am so struck by his behaviour is disturbing. When a doctor does his or her job is this a miracle? Throughout my course of treatment I have had both 'good' and 'bad' doctors. The good, who have been the majority, have acted justly and respectfully; the bad, haphazardly and with disrespect (meanness?). My experience with this first doctor was good, and for this I am thankful.

bone marrow aspiration—made diagnosis much easier than it often is. Frequently, doctors are faced with an unorganized series of vague, recurrent, changing signs that are described subjectively (Brown, 1995). The doctor even has to trust that these various signs, normal as some might be (a pain in the knee, tiredness, loss of appetite), are legitimately outside of the normal experience of the person and that the complaint should be taken seriously.

Most illnesses that general practitioners and family doctors confront in their everyday work are self-limiting and minor—colds, flu, and bacterial infections. Some people go to the doctor for social and emotional support; others for help with psychosomatic symptoms. Life-threatening illnesses are not routine—even in the work of the doctor. About 910 children under the age of 15 are diagnosed with cancer in Canada yearly (McBride, 1998), while about 57,000 doctors were practising in Canada in 1997 (IMS Health Strategic Technologies, 1999; see also Clarke, 1996: 265). Clearly, most doctors never get to see and diagnose a case of childhood cancer—let alone leukemia, which though the most frequent is not the only childhood cancer—in a number of years of practice.

In a similar story, the 21-year-old son of sociologist Alexandra Todd was diagnosed in 1991 with a 'fast growing, aggressive, large tumor in the sphenoid sinus area of the head' after being sick for over a year with various vague symptoms (Todd, 1994: 2). During the year before his diagnosis he was tested and treated for a wildly varying number of diseases, including mononucleosis, dairy allergies, eczema, impetigo, extreme dry skin, cluster headaches, stress, and flu. He visited a variety of specialists and had a battery of tests, including a CAT scan and even a complete workup at Stanford Medical Center. Finally, he went to an ophthalmologist, who knew that something serious might be wrong and made an immediate referral to a neurologist. Within a couple of weeks there was an answer and a serious diagnosis.

Todd has written about the various normalizing efforts of all involved. Her son Drew slept all day and woke just to go to class, do his homework, or have a bit to eat. His girlfriend compensated. She shook him awake to go to class and brought him food from the school cafeteria. His mother and stepfather encouraged him to eliminate dairy foods (as this had helped his mother in a dramatic manner previously); his father arranged for testing at Stanford but lived across the country and couldn't observe his ongoing health struggles. The local family physician thought he was just stressed by exams. Again, a serious life-threatening diagnosis began with recurrent and changing symptoms that were subjectively defined. The infrequency of a diagnosis of childhood cancer adds to the tendency we have as human beings, parents, sufferers, and even, at times, doctors to normalize extreme changes and then make the typical diagnosis process lengthy.

A study of 33 Midwestern US families whose children were diagnosed with cancer reported that none of the parents, when they observed the symptoms in their children, believed that there was a serious problem:

> All parents indicated that they had never considered the possibility that their child's symptoms represented a serious illness. Although they were aware that something was wrong, they used a familiar, non-threatening, explanatory framework to interpret the child's symptoms. They had assumed that the problem was minor or relatively common; a persistent respiratory infection, diarrhea, a reaction to immunization, an insect bite, crossed eyes, appendicitis or something similar. (Martinson and Cohen, 1988: 84)

Sociologists have found that a useful way of describing the relationship between symptom observation and medically relevant action is as an iceberg. Most of an iceberg is under water—very little is observed by passing ships, by telescope, or by the naked eye. Similarly, most illness is suffered at home, at work, and on the playground. Most of the time people do not go to the doctor with various signs and symptoms but expect that they will take care of themselves and will disappear in the face of a concerted effort to have extra sleep, eat particularly well, and, in general ways, take health-promotion dictates seriously, at least for a time. 'Normalization' of unusual symptoms is, well, normal.

All of us, doctors and others, including present and future patients, live in the world of the 'taken-for-granted'. Our worlds are enmeshed in what we take to be normal. 'The individuals' common sense knowledge of the world is a system of constructs of its typicality' (Schutz, 1967: 7). We all assume that what was essentially the case yesterday remains the case today and will be so into the future. Our lives are enmeshed in norms. We mostly interact with others and ourselves through a common language, with common etiquette and other rules for behaviour. As a teacher at university, I am always impressed that students who are free to sit wherever they choose in class almost always select the same seat in the same row, week after week, through the term. At least one colleague has suggested that the location in class is often connected with grades. Those at the front are most likely to receive A's. I'm not sure about this connection to grades, but the norm of territoriality is seldom violated. It is no wonder, then, that illness is often normalized both by the ill and by those in the business of noticing and labelling illness.

My reaction to the changing pot-pourri of symptoms reflects my background and my reality. I have myself generally felt quite healthy and, aside from the removal of tonsils when I was about five and the births of my two daughters, I have largely been able to avoid allopathic medicine and its practitioners. (Allopathic medicine is the currently hegemonic paradigm of professionalized medicine in our society, with a focus on licensed physicians, hospitals, prescription drugs, and curing specific invasive illnesses and healing particular wounds, as opposed, for example, to a focus on the whole person.) As a medical sociologist I had learned to be questioning about the truth and value of allopathic medicine and its evidence base. As an educated, middle-class, sort of left-wing woman who has been involved since the early days of the women's health movement in a more or less informed critique of medical dominance, I had many questions. I had questioned the 'medicalization of childbirth' when I had been pregnant with my daughters and read all I could about 'natural' childbirth, midwifery, the LeBoyer method of immersing the baby in water after birth, and other topics related to natural birth. Had it been possible at the time I would have used a midwife during the pregnancies and deliveries. My goal was to have as 'natural' a childbirth as possible. This essentially meant, at the time, to avoid doctors, hospital, drugs, and surgery to the extent that I was able. (In the end, I gave birth by Caesarean section. But that is another story.)

I had taken my daughters to allopathic doctors when I felt their conditions warranted intervention, which was, for me, as for many others, when their symptoms were acute and I supposed that they might need an antibiotic. My general approach to illness was based on typical explanatory frameworks, as Kleinman (1988: 121) puts it:

> Explanatory models are the notions that patients, families and practitioners have about a specific illness episode. They respond to such questions as: What is the nature of this problem? Why has it affected me? Why now? What course will it follow? How does it affect my body? What treatment do I deserve? What do I most fear about this illness and its treatment? Explanatory models are responses to urgent life circumstances.

They also reflect aspects of the dominant health discourses.

Prevention and health promotion are two such discourses that have been widely espoused and even endorsed by international and national government bodies in the last quarter of the twentieth century. In 1974 Marc Lalonde, the Minister of Health in the Canadian federal government, published a book called *A New Perspective on the Health of Canadians*, in which he argued for a broadening of health concerns to include a consideration of factors in addition to biology, including environmental and lifestyle factors. In 1986 the federal government, this time under the imprimatur of Health Minister Jake Epp, published another guidebook for reconceptualizing health, *Achieving Health for All: A Framework for Health Promotion*. Again, it served to broaden the focus of health beyond biology to include mechanisms for preventing and addressing health problems, such as self-care, mutual aid, and the development of healthy environments. These health promotion and prevention discourses have achieved national and international acclaim and have permeated Canadian health policies of the latter part of the twentieth century. It is probably no wonder, then, that as a citizen of Canada today, I first turned to prevention and health promotion as explanatory frameworks for my daughter's symptoms. And when I became truly concerned, spinach and raisins were the menu.

The other framework to which I turned is also culturally dominant. This is the tendency to individualize medical problems and to look for psychological explanations and solutions (Waitzkin, 1989). This perspective is consistent with the contemporary rejection of Descartes's split between the mind and the body by an alternative model that holds that the body and the mind are one. In medicine and medical research this tendency has been translated into the new science of psychoneuroimmunology, a 'field of study that investigates the interactions between the neuroendocrine and immune systems in response to environmental circumstances and the psychological factors that mediate these interactions' (Caudell, 1996: 493). This can be seen in my explanations to myself of Lauren's tiredness as being related to her experience of loss—of her two best friends (one for a year and the other for a month), of her favourite teacher and mentor who retired the previous June—and her disappointment at her electoral defeat when she had run for school president the previous year, rather than, for instance, an environmental carcinogen such as a pesticide.

My suggestion that I turned to health promotion, disease prevention, and social-psychological explanations is not necessarily a self-criticism. There are times when these strategies work as they are intended. The more that we understand, the more evidence is accumulating about the promise and contribution to health of psychoneuroimmunology. Disease prevention and health promotion have great potential for the well-being of whole populations. Obviously, though, such preoccupations may encourage us to ignore early symptoms of serious illness.

CHAPTER 2

CHOREOGRAPHING AND TELLING THE DIAGNOSIS

Lauren and I drove from Kitchener to the big city hospital, picking up my sister, Cindy, on the way. We had been told not to wait in the hospital waiting room but to ask to go immediately into the emergency ward. This didn't really sink in. So when we arrived I went to the desk and explained that Suzi had made arrangements for Lauren to be admitted to the pediatric ward. They were confused behind the desk and didn't have any information. So we went back to sit in the waiting room. But my sister reminded me that Suzi had said not to wait in the waiting room and so I went back to the desk to explain. (We later found out that we were not to stay in the waiting room because Lauren's neutrophil counts were so low that she did not have any resistance—if there were people with contagious diseases in the waiting room Lauren could pick up the 'germs'. (The neutrophils are the most numerous of the granulocytic white cells, the function of which is to move through the bloodstream to defend the body against bacteria, viruses, and some type of fungus.)

This time we were taken to a small room in the emergency wing with a curtain over its door. It all seemed surreal. Lauren felt well enough. She had been tired for a while and reported being very tired at times. But we are all tired at times. What were these mysterious blood counts and why were they so important? Why was Lauren able to sit, talk, and visit with her Aunt Cindy without any signs of suffering? Neither Lauren nor I believed that anything could really be 'the matter'.

The pediatric hemotology resident doctor was paged and within an hour or so a very pretty, very young, and very friendly woman came and introduced herself. She proceeded to examine Lauren and then to ask questions. Certain questions stand out! She asked if there was any cancer in the family and I had to say that my mother had both a brother and a sister die of cancer when they were young children, about six years old. I had heard many stories of Ann and Sonny over the years. I'd heard how they both died in Grandma's arms; how Grandpa 'lost everything' as he travelled from country to country to find a cure for his only son, Sonny, in a family of nine daughters; how Sonny's cancer had been discovered by a barber who noticed a lump behind his ear. I remembered the pictures of both of the children laid out in their coffins—Ann's velvet dress and Sonny in breeches and a fine dress shirt. Several of my mother's other sisters had cancer as adults—one had recently died. There was other cancer, too, on my dad's side of the family—skin cancer, in this case, but it was not the life-threatening kind. There was some cancer, but less, and in any case less known to me, in Lauren's dad's family.

Next the doctor tried to eliminate drugs as a cause for Lauren's blood counts, and she could. Lauren had not used any drugs but vitamin C, which we had always used when 'under the weather', and echinacea, a newer herb from the roots of the purple coneflower, a recently popularized immune-system builder. The doctor had never heard of echinacea. This should not have been surprising to me as it was the darling of the alternative health industry and had been for a few years. It was not, however, a mainstream prescription drug.

I asked what she was looking for and trying to eliminate—what was the differential diagnosis? And when she said leukemia or aplastic anemia, I leapt on aplastic anemia, not knowing what it was but believing that it could be treated with iron. Little did I realize that leukemia was the better of the two diseases because there is a more effective (usually) treatment for it. Aplastic anemia, on the other hand, I learned later, was essentially untreatable without a bone marrow transplant. And that involves finding a donor—in a situation where the odds may be very steep indeed—and then living through the transplant, the anti-rejection drugs, and all the associated side-effects. But I didn't know any of this at the time and so I held on to the hope that it must be aplastic anemia or a mistaken lab test. When I try to think of how I felt at the time, the closest that I can get to it is 'on guard'. I was like a guard dog except that, rather than showing my teeth, I was trying to be and appear to be helpful, informed, and intelligent. I wanted to appear knowledgeable and reasonable. Did I believe that this would protect Lauren? Probably. I was being a 'good mother'. 'Good mothers' don't let bad things happen to their children. If I was a 'good mother' perhaps the whole thing would be a mistake. Lab tests could be wrong.[1]

After a number of hours Lauren was admitted and taken upstairs on a hospital gurney. I walked along beside her. I cannot remember this from the inside. I can only visualize myself walking along beside my daughter, 'on guard' and in shock. We were admitted to a blue room on the pediatric medical floor, and Lauren was put on an intravenous antibiotic. The nurse gave her mouthwashes. It seemed a bit odd. She said 'they'll want you to take these.' She explained to Lauren that one was a 'swish and a swallow' and the other a 'swish and spit'. Mouthwashes raised alarm bells in me (which were quickly suppressed) because I knew that mouth sores were a side-effect of chemotherapy and that mouthwashes were given as a prevention.

The nurse, without being explicit, seemed to know what was wrong with Lauren. The fact that this nurse seemed to know what Lauren's diagnosis was, or at least was likely to be, did not permit her to mention it. Nor did I ever consider asking because the rules of telling are such firm rules (Sudnow, 1967). Eventually, we got to sleep. I slept on the chair in Lauren's single room. It longitudinally folded over into a short bed. The sleep was short and fitful until the hospital got busy in the morning at about 6 or 7 a.m.

The evening before, prior to leaving home, I had called Lauren's stepmother, Marian, to tell her that we were on our way to the hospital and briefly explained what had happened over the day to lead to this. I told Marian that I would call her and Richard, Lauren's dad, later. Richard was at work and occupied until after 9 p.m. that evening and so I knew that I would not be able to speak with him until then. Around 10:30 I had called and explained the situation to

---

1 I, too, thought that aplastic anemia sounded plausible, almost positive. All I needed were some iron supplements, a little rest, and perhaps a reduction in course and school activities. These changes would cure me.

Richard and then called Jess, Lauren's older sister, a third-year student at university, to tell her that Lauren was in the hospital and that we'd call whenever there was news about what was wrong.[2] Wednesday morning Richard and Marion arrived early—probably 9 or 10. My sister made arrangements for the care of her three children and arrived at the hospital, too. Lauren and I were moved to the pediatric hematology ward, to another single room.

Fortunately, I thought at the time, I have insurance, and extended benefits that provided for a single hospital room. Later, I discovered that the single room was medically necessary because of Lauren's vulnerable condition. She was, we learned, neutropenic, which meant that her neutrophil white blood cell count was so low that she was extremely vulnerable to infection and had virtually no resistance. The single room was imperative.

Once we were moved, another resident came by with the pediatric hematologist to do a bone marrow aspiration. This was the test we were all waiting for. Cloths and trays, slides and tubes, and needles and bigger needles arrived. Nurses and lab technicians gathered around the bed ready to run the bone marrow to the lab for testing.[3] Time stopped, and it seemed that everyone stopped breathing—until the doctor laid out her tools and began to explain what she was going to do. She was to go into Lauren's lower back with a needle, which was to be inserted into a bone in an area where there was generally a lot of accessible marrow. I had heard horror stories of the pain involved. However Lauren hadn't and I just couldn't believe that they could be true.

The situation quickly became ritualized. The resident doctor announced that she was going to do the bone marrow aspiration. And then Richard, who had been sitting next to Lauren, moved back

---

2 I asked Mom to tell my dad and Marion not to come down. It would have meant an hour's drive late at night for what I felt was nothing. In the morning I would be told I was fine, just anemic, and I would go home. There was no possibility that I could be sick.

3 It is odd to me now that they performed this test in my hospital room. It is their policy never to do a painful procedure in the child's room (except IV and finger poke insertions, which in time grew to be very painful). They refrain from this because they do not want the child to associate pain with her or his living space. However, in an effort not to increase the tension around this act they (and I) did it in my room.

so I could sit close and hold her hand. Cindy sat near me with the lunch menu for the next day, then Richard and then Marian. Our seating arrangements were a clue to the dynamics of intimacy: Lauren and I closest, then her dad; my sister close to me, but on my other side; Marian was as close to Richard, but on his other side. The rules of intimacy may be unwritten but they are rigorous, nevertheless.

It hurt. It really hurt. Lauren had tears in her eyes. She was wincing. The resident was having a hard time. The procedure is difficult. It requires accuracy and physical strength. She tried twice and then gave up—I think she, too, had tears in her eyes.[4] Full of apologies, she asked the senior doctor, with many years' experience, to do it. People from the lab came up and stood at the end of the bed. The experienced hemotologist, after applying even more of the substance used to anesthetize the skin with what appeared to be lots and lots of 'freezing', asked her to curl up in the fetal position, got the bone marrow out with apparent ease, and filled what seemed at the time to be about 20 vials with the substance.

All the while, whenever there was a moment's break, Cindy joked about the food and read the menu to Lauren. The choices were not exactly appealing. Lauren was a vegetarian, and a teenager with very specific and limited eating habits. So playing around—do you want white bread with butter or without butter?—seemed funny, silly, and ludicrous, and in between the painful moments we all laughed.[5] That was that, medically. We were told they would have the diagnosis that afternoon. In the afternoon, the resident and the experienced doctor came back to say that they had the results but

---

4   This resident became one of my favourites. She would come in and chat with me and Mom. She would actually give me a full physical, rather than the cursory one I became used to with other residents. She would listen to my questions and complaints. Through her actions she made me feel safe and taken care of. Part of the reason she may have had difficulty working on my back was that I was a fully grown woman and she was used to working on children. My back was a lot bigger than her norm. The pain I remember cognitively as being a lot. However, our bodies have the wonderful ability to let us forget the actual feeling of pain, and thankfully I have.

5   I have many happy memories from those long-ago hospital days. One of my fondest is Cindy's humorous recital during that painful day. I love food and to picture chocolate pudding and French fries—foods I normally did not eat—was fun and distracting. Cindy saved that procedure as much as the experienced doctor did.

didn't want to tell us until they had them confirmed and had more information, unless we wanted the preliminary details. We declined. We called Jess and asked her to come the next day to be there for the diagnosis. The next day Jess arrived and Cindy and I went out to meet her. It was the last time I left the hospital for about three weeks. Then, I was still trying to pretend to myself that I wasn't worried and wanted to meet Jess to reassure her that everyone was okay.

Shortly after we got back the doctors arrived at our room. They asked if Richard and I, as the parents, wanted to hear the news first and then tell Lauren. We instantly agreed that we should all be present.[6] Later, as I reviewed the literature I found that our immediate and intuitive response was probably the one with the greatest support in the research literature on pediatric oncology. As one article put it: 'a number of carefully controlled studies provide convincing evidence for the rationale of the open approach' (Van Dongen-Melman and Sanders-Woudstra, 1986: 147). It is important for children to know as much as they can about the disease and its treatment from the very beginning. If they do not know as a result of being formally included in honest discussion, then they imagine (and usually imagine 'the worst') or find out informally (see Bluebond-Langer, 1978, for a detailed description of how children learn their own diagnosis, the varieties of treatment available, and other such things, even when they are not told).

Once again we found our places. I held Lauren's hand and sat up close to her head where I could touch her and listen. Marian chose a place outside the circle of Lauren, Jess, her dad, and me. Cindy was again close but outside the immediate circle. The doctor said they had all the tests back and confirmed by a hospital lab downtown and, I believe, by one in the United States, and that Lauren had acute lymphoblastic leukemia (ALL). The doctor then very quickly assured us that she had the 'good' kind of leukemia

---

6   I am glad that I heard it at first, too. I was 17, old enough to make many decisions on my own. I was also asked who else could be there. I wanted Jess and Marian and Cindy to all be present. I felt that we were all in it together by this point and that 'something big' was about to be revealed.

and that her prognosis for full recovery was 78–82 per cent.[7] He added that theirs was the very best treatment protocol in the world, except one in Germany that seemed to be 1 or 2 percentage points better. And Lauren had the good kind of cells—there were two possibilities and she had the better kind. Though the distinction between types of cells is one that we never did come to understand, we both remember the doctor making the distinction. In fact, he said, a woman in her thirties, who had had this disease years ago had just come to see him with her three kids.[8]

The treatment was based on a protocol developed at and supervised from a hospital in the United States, and there were a number of hospitals in the US and Canada in this protocol. He said the treatment should begin the next day with remission induction, i.e., chemotherapy to (hopefully) induce remission of the disease, and then, when asked, he said that treatment would be about two years in duration. All of this was presented as positive information—his report was so upbeat. He was aware, as we weren't, of all of the much poorer diagnoses and prognoses there might have been. The information was portrayed optimistically and encouragingly. Lauren said, either then or very shortly after, 'I'm not 78, or 80–82 per cent, I'm 100 per cent! In other words, she was sure that she was going to 'make it'. The doctors then left the room and said they would wait outside while we talked, in case we had more questions. After maybe another half-hour to an hour we invited them back in and asked a number of questions about the treatment protocol, about the withdrawal from the protocol, about the willingness to change the treatment if it was not working, about how frequently Lauren would receive treatment. They answered the questions, we signed, and Lauren, because she was 17, signed, too, agreeing to take part in the study treatment.

---

7   It didn't happen quite as quickly as this account portrays. In my memory we had all just gotten our lunches and were starting to eat. The air in the room felt almost festive to me; however, this feeling was in reality a high level of anxiety and denial on my part. These were, after all, my last 'free' moments for the next two years.

8   This doctor was always highly positive. He saw me as a person, and I think a little like his daughter, and wanted me to be as normal as possible. He pushed for my early release from hospital, not wanting to disrupt my life.

It was an amazing experience, so tightly choreographed that we felt optimistic and, if not relieved, then ultimately hopeful about a

> **Living With Cancer**
>
> What were you doing on 12 October 1995? It was the Thursday just after Thanksgiving of that year. Maybe you were handing in papers to professors or teachers. Maybe you had a cold and were lying in your residence, trying to down the orange juice your roommate had so graciously picked up for you at Brubaker's. Maybe you have no recollection of that day. I do.
>
> That was the day I sat on a hospital bed surrounded by my family at a large teaching hospital. At noon that day I heard for the first time why I had been tired and lacking in strength and energy that summer and the first month of grade twelve. This was also when I learned a little about what would consume the next two years of my life.
>
> My doctors told me that I had been diagnosed, after blood tests and a bone marrow test, with acute lymphoblastic leukemia: cancer of the blood. My doctors were quick to inform me that the disease had been caught early. It was the 'easiest' leukemia to deal with and it had a higher than 80 per cent survival rate. These were great signs. All in all, things couldn't have been better under the circumstances.
>
> I received my first massive chemotherapy dose the next morning. What started so abruptly is a process that I am still living through. Now, almost a tenth of my life has been spent in treatment. I receive steroids and other drugs that, while poisoning and killing my good, healthy powerful cells, are also saving me.
>
> It is amazing to me that so much of my life has been so 'normal' the past two years and yet this shadow, this elephant, has been consistently walking beside me, and at times, nudging me from my path to go off and graze.
>
> Cancer is not a disease that newborns, children, or young adults are supposed to get. Neither is cancer an illness that adults and seniors should have to deal with. It kills, maims, and hurts the millions who receive the diagnosis.
>
> It also has an enormous impact on these individuals' support networks. My family has been walking this path with me, sometimes in more

> fear and pain than I. Some of my friends have not known what to do or say, and some have pulled through in ways that still keep me warm....
>
> From *Imprint* (University of Waterloo), 26 Sept. 1997

treatment that would work and return Lauren to good health. I have often wondered about the significance for our subsequent coping of the way we were told. The doctor was so reassuring and normalizing. He answered all of our questions. He emphasized that the treatment was one of the best in the world. There were ways out of this particular treatment if we changed our minds. He was respectful of Lauren, who was in an unusual situation as a 17-year-old. She was already an adult in many ways. She could legally drive a car, for instance. Yet she still technically fit into the classification of pediatrics. I am often grateful that the doctor who gave the diagnosis was who he was. He was kind. He listened. And the hope he offered was often the cushion upon which my fearful head rested. It was the energy that I sometimes needed to run up and down stairs to do the laundry. It provided the courage I needed to talk to all the assembled teachers at Lauren's high school about her situation and about how we expected them to respond. It provided a backdrop of hope as Lauren underwent the terrible treatments in the next months and years.

Three aspects of this experience have been the subject of research and reflection by social scientists. These include reactions to an illness diagnosis, the role of hope, and the choreographing of the announcement of the diagnosis.

What is the effect of learning a diagnosis? Was it a relief to us to know what was wrong, finally?[9] Was the diagnosis devastating? Certainly it was an awful shock. Yet the preliminaries, including the call from the doctor at the urgent-care clinic on Tuesday; the differential diagnoses mentioned by the resident on Tuesday night; the

---

9   I have to say that it was not a relief, for I didn't really feel ill. There I went from being a super-involved though a little tired student to a cancer patient, all in a few hours. That was not the ending I was expecting. This was not my diagnosis.

mouthwashes; the seriousness of the bone marrow aspiration; the fact of being in hospital; and the sombre remarks of the doctor on Wednesday afternoon after the initial lab results, that they had a diagnosis that wasn't confirmed or complete but would be the next day—all of these clues to an extent prepared us. I cannot remember feeling the 'horror' of what was one of the worst things I could imagine happening in my life. The diagnosis, and our awareness of its seriousness, had inevitably been incremental.

The relevant literature on this topic is quite variable. In some studies the diagnosis is experienced as a relief. It is felt to be the final end in a long and confusing search to understand and find a meaning for an uncomfortable, painful, or otherwise unusual way of feeling. Diseases such as multiple sclerosis, lupus, chronic fatigue syndrome, and Alzheimer's disease are examples where diagnosis of the multiple, changing, and often troubling symptoms is often experienced as a relief, for the diagnosis has frequently been preceded by a long search for explanation, for understanding. Finally, sufferers report, someone believes and takes them seriously. At last, someone has heard and believed their stories about changing body experiences. Now, they report feeling, something can be done (Brown, 1995).

Other studies suggest that the diagnosis makes the sufferer sicker. Realizing what it is that is wrong and receiving medical legitimization for it make the experience worse. Such has been thought to be the case with such diagnoses as a heart attack or cancer. Here, it is said, the meaning of the diagnosis in itself leads the sufferer to feel sicker than he or she might otherwise have felt (Clarke, 1985).[10]

What was the case in my situation? The diagnosis was a shock. I had no idea at all that Lauren had a life-threatening illness. I did not realize or understand what the tiredness Lauren said she felt was like. She had carried on with all her regular school, extracurricular, and social activities. She seemed happy. She was full of plans

---

10 In the case of cancer, it seems that the medicine is much worse than the initial illness. Yes, one would (does) suffer terribly from later stages of cancer, but in my case tiredness and lights in my eyes were nothing compared to the nausea and pain of chemotherapy and radiation.

and had just finished a newspaper to welcome grade nine students to her school and was organizing a 30-hour 'famine' put on by students to raise money for development projects in the 'developing world'. She said she was tired. But I, like the doctors who have a difficult time acting on subjective reports of pain and fatigue (Brown, 1995), did not comprehend the serious nature of Lauren's complaint. Thus my shock at the realization of how serious this symptom (of tiredness) really was.

I don't remember feeling; instead, I remember planning the actions that had to be taken. I remember thinking, okay, that's it, now what do we do? Interestingly to me now, the only thoughts I had about actions that were to be taken had to do with telling other people. I hadn't eaten for a few days but I wasn't hungry. I had just brought one nightie and a change of underwear, but I was not concerned about having either clean or different clothes to wear. I had a full-time job and although I was on a fellowship leave I still had research and teaching assistants (for my distance education courses) to supervise, a book due at the publisher within a few months, meetings, and a social life. None of this came to mind. My concern was focused on the immediate tasks that lay ahead: telling others; packing our things so we could move to a treatment room; Lauren's needs, for friends, books, music, and the like.

I guess that is shock. That Lauren would not live never entered my mind at this point. I, too, was sure 'she was 100 per cent'. She seemed so healthy, except for the tiredness, and we had a course of action that, taken step by step, would lead to a return to good health. I do remember being shocked by learning the length of treatment and about the requirement of weekly hospital visits for chemotherapy. Yet, even the length and arduousness of this process did not really hit me at this time.

There has been a lot of discussion about the positive benefits of hope. Its importance for helping people to 'emotionally endure crisis' and significant difficulties of various sorts has been described. What remains unclear, however, is what encourages, establishes, and maintains hope for people in various situations. Specifically, current literature does not clearly define the particular components of the patient-doctor interaction that assist in the establishment and continuance of hope. Wong-Wylie and Jevne (1997) have begun to address this lack through lengthy and detailed interviews with people with HIV or AIDS. Their respondents were asked to discuss incidents in their interactions with their doctors that led to increased or decreased hope.

They found that those with whom they spoke described their experiences with hope and hopelessness in ways that could be organized into five paired factors of opposing valences: (1) being known as a human being as compared to being known as a case; (2) feeling connected to or having rapport with the doctor or not; (3) doctors being descriptive and outlining choices as compared to giving orders and direction; (4) feeling welcomed by doctors who were or tried to be accessible as compared with experiencing the doctors as always being in a hurry; and (5) perceiving that the doctor was providing up-to-date information, on one hand, or giving little or inadequate information, on the other. What all of this means is what you might expect—patients would rather be known as persons than diseases, like to feel human connection, prefer to believe they have choices, like to be given the time they need to be heard, and, finally, like to be informed. It is not that excellent medical care at the very best treatment centres offered by the very best doctors is not valued. It is. Technical competence, perhaps because of the professional and financial status of doctors, is assumed. Patients tend to want to take that for granted. In addition to this, though, patients and families want their own humanity, and that of the medical personnel, to be recognized. This is the simple arithmetic: one plus one equals good care.

One other striking feature of the experience of the diagnosis was the physical placement of each of us in relation to the others. Sudnow (1967) observed two different hospitals in the United States over a period of about two years, particularly focusing on how death occurred, was handled, talked about, and announced. He noted how some but not other events that occur in hospital are considered to be 'announceable' events. Everyone, he found, knew what these events were. 'A sudden turn for the worse, the outcome of a surgical procedure, the result of a child delivery' (1967: 117) are examples of such occurrences. Not only, however, did certain events demand announcement, but clearly specified people were 'responsible' for their announcement. In general, the more important and serious the event the more likely the doctor would be the designated announcer. Certain questions were to be answered by the doctor and only by the doctor.

Most announceable events, Sudnow found, were embedded in a 'specifically structured episode' and with a particular organization of talk. For example, when 'news' is being announced, it is not embedded in a long conversation or even a short conversation about the weather, the score of the hockey game, or a recipe for Thanksgiving turkey. If the news is 'it's a boy', that news comes first in the conversation and then 'small talk' may follow. The announcer's demeanour and tone are also expected to reflect and to be consistent with the message being given. A smile and a happy voice are appropriate to good news. A serious face and a sombre voice are appropriate to bad news. When there might be some doubt about the news, the announcer may be likely to appear in professional garb—in a lab coat, surgical scrubs—and to carry other props that reflect the authority that is (hopefully) being portrayed. Thus are announcements tightly scripted, choreographed, and, just as in a good stage play, the sets, costumes, and the tone of dialogue are carefully predetermined.

Sudnow describes how the announcement of a serious medical condition follows certain very clearly defined steps. He calls these announcement rules 'the family roll call' and suggests that they provide an 'occasion' for drawing the boundaries of the social unit. Our experience demonstrates how the process of drawing family boundaries, and, I would add, reinforcing family structure through elaboration of what might be called the 'hierarchies of intimacy', was relevant in carrying out the serious, determinative procedure of the bone marrow aspiration, as well as the announcement of the diagnosis. Such rules, it should be noted, are relevant not only to the announcement of 'bad' news but also to 'good' news. For example, the announcement of an upcoming marriage or birth of a child follows and reinforces family structures of intimacy. These rules are to be taken seriously. Their violation constitutes a breach of the normative order.

The order of telling mirrors the order of closeness in the kinship lineage and friendship network. Thus, the immediate family is followed by more distant family and by friends. Furthermore, depending on the degree of closeness, certain strategies are warranted. It would not be considered appropriate, in most cases, to inform the immediate family of a serious change in an individual family member by letter, although exceptions might be made in the case of long distance or the unavailability of a telephone. The immediate family is believed to be entitled to know in a speedy and direct fashion. Moreover, the order of telling is ordained to move along the chain of intimacy. It would not be appropriate for a more distant family member to hear the news before a closer family member. Such are the rules of announcement of diagnosis and related news.[11] We followed these unwritten rules both in the immediate moments of the bone marrow aspiration and in the time of the actual diagnosis.

When I think about it now I wonder why we did not seek a second opinion. We live in a densely populated area of Ontario and there are three pediatric oncology centres at almost equal distance from our home. I had studied medical sociology and I knew that it was often advisable to get a second and even third opinion, especially in the case of a serious illness. Even the American Medical Association recommends that patients seek a second opinion prior to consenting to any invasive procedures (Keene, 1997: 121). Many insurance companies in the US require second opinions. Nevertheless, whether because of shock, denial, fear, exhaustion, inability to think, or some other odd dynamic, we thought only briefly about the possibility of seeking a second opinion. I wonder if it was the personal warmth of the doctor coupled with his confidence in the protocol that led us all to want to leap to trust him and the treatment he was offering. In our shock and virtually absolute ignorance about childhood cancer and its treatment options, I suppose we wanted to act immediately

---

11 When I was diagnosed I needed to tell my closest friends, Meaghan and Mike, about my illness myself. I also wanted a few of my closer friends and teachers to be called and told before they heard the news at school. Making sure that others were okay was very important to me.

to get rid of this awful problem. We wanted someone who knew how to take care of it. And the diagnosing doctor appeared perfectly suited at the time.

CHAPTER 3

ACKNOWLEDGING THE DIAGNOSIS, TELLING OTHERS, AND THINKING ABOUT CAUSATION

Almost immediately, even urgently, after we heard the diagnosis we seemed to need to tell certain other people. This seemed to have the significance of a news bulletin. The world had altered. It had moved. Our world had completely changed during the past few hours. Lauren had changed irrevocably.[1] Her life and ours—her sister, parents, and stepmother's lives—would be changed. Who to tell? When? Where? What? We quickly decided that since it was Lauren's news primarily, telling her friends was a priority. Richard and Marian and I privately decided how and when to tell our immediate family members.

Since my sister, Cindy, was there, we discussed how to divide the labour of telling family and my closest friends. Actually, she did all of the telling. I knew I couldn't inform people close to me and be coherent at the same time. I wasn't crying but I was holding on to my strength by a very slim string. I spoke with her about calling my brother, who was halfway across the country in Halifax. We decided just to warn him that Lauren was sick and in the hospital but not to tell him the diagnosis. We decided to leave telling my mother and my other sister, who was less involved in the family, until later. I couldn't even face calling my mother. I could not face her worries or questions. My role as the eldest child was being one of my widowed and elderly mother's supporters and I knew I didn't have the emotional energy to fulfil my expectations about how I should relate to her at this time. My other sister lived a life that was fairly independent of mine and so calling her immediately seemed less important.

There was a party the next night with my department colleagues

---

[1] This is a difficult statement for me to accept. I believe that everything that happens to us, and every choice we make, changes us. This one fact, that I had cancer, is not the most important change in my life. It is one event that helps form me, but not more than that.

in honour of one of the department's secretaries, who was retiring. I was expected, but I knew that it was not necessary either that I be there or that I call to explain. I was on a research leave for the year, having won a national fellowship for a study on the politicization of breast cancer. I was also very lucky that I did not have classes to teach, as I know that I would have been in a terrible dilemma about whether or not I would be able to get back to the classroom. I had a speaking engagement at which I was to accept the fellowship in Montreal the following week: I asked my sister to call and cancel. I knew I wouldn't be able to talk to an outsider. I was doing all I could to manage my emotions within the hospital and with the hospital personnel.

Cindy and I decided to ask our brother to drive up and tell our mother in person. We also planned that as soon as he told her he would offer to bring her down to the hospital to see Lauren. He did and she came and stood outside the door, with one of her old nurse's masks on, in case she had germs. She brought a dozen or so home-made butter tarts for Lauren, as they were one of Lauren's favourite treats.

Lauren decided that there were two people she wanted and needed to tell right away. Their lives were tied up with hers. We called and asked Meaghan, her best friend of over three years, and Michael, Lauren's boyfriend for more than two years, to come down to the hospital so that Lauren could explain what had happened. We planned that we would all leave the room so that she could tell Michael and Meaghan alone.[2] The order of telling was rigidly organized, just as the seating arrangements when the bone marrow aspiration was done and the diagnosis was given. Unwritten, yet clear and firm rules directed our behaviours.

Michael's parents drove down to the hospital with Mike and Meaghan. Richard, Jess, Marian, and I went to the parents' room and talked with them. Richard's sister and her husband drove over from a nearby city and so they, too, were in the parents' room. We talked about all the good news: it was not AML (acute myelogenic

---

2   They brought me a beautiful bouquet of red and yellow roses. I could tell they were nervous. In fact, later I found out that one of my teachers had asked Mike if I had leukemia before we even knew. Mike had looked up information about this unknown disease. The information had been out of date and thus Mike was scared.

leukemia), which we had now learned was much more difficult to treat, but ALL; we had a great doctor and a great treatment protocol; and Lauren's prognosis from the doctor was hopeful, as was her own 100 per cent assessment. We emphasized the positives. There really was no part of me that expected, at this time, that Lauren would not 'make it'. Okay, she had leukemia ... but that wasn't really so bad. It was treatable and the prognosis was good. She still seemed well enough. She was tired, as she had been before the diagnosis, but otherwise all the other signs of physical abnormalities, such as bruising, enlarged spleen, and recurrent or continuous high fever, were absent. She was fully conscious and we were all around her. Nothing really bad could happen. We were still coping by being optimistic. The diagnosing doctor had offered hope and optimism. Lauren had topped his optimism. I mirrored this optimism. Everything was going to work out.

There were a number of questions we asked at the time—we were curious about the causes of ALL, about the length and effectiveness of the treatment. We were not really yet concerned about side-effects, long-term effects, or after-effects. We were not looking ahead in a realistic way. Time was eclipsed, yet interminable. Instead, we put our trust totally in the doctors, nurses, and the hospital. We believed at that time that 'they' knew best, that 'they' had all of the answers and the way to a complete cure. After all, this was reputed to be an excellent hospital and the research treatment protocol was tied into other excellent, major university-affiliated hospitals. There was no need to question this hospital, this doctor, or this treatment, was there?

Lauren did ask a doctor if she was sure, and how she was sure, that she had leukemia. She wanted to know what the distinguishing characteristics of her blood were. She wanted to make sure there was no mistake. One of the pediatric oncologists (who left the hospital to move to another city almost immediately after Lauren's diagnosis) arranged for Lauren to go with her to the hemotology lab to see some blood samples. This doctor showed Lauren, in a microscope in the lab on the first floor of the hospital, what her blood looked like, what leukemia cells, red and white blood cells, and platelets looked like.

Lauren also very quickly wanted to use her experience to be a help to others. She asked what was known about cause and said that she would be happy to be part of any research that was examining cancer causation. The diagnosing doctor responded that there was a large epidemiological study under way in Canada, but added that it was asking so many questions that it would be useless. I gathered that a study reporting a higher incidence of childhood cancer associated with exposure to electromagnetic rays (such as electric blankets and electricity towers) had recently been reported because several of the doctors dismissed this study in casual conversations about causation.

But we were interested in cause. We wanted to understand what had happened to lead to this totally unexpected diagnosis. We are, as humans, used to taking our worlds, our friendships, our families and bodies for granted. Yet our common-sense thinking is causal. We learn to predict our lives through a myriad of smaller and larger signs. Grey clouds often bring rain or snow. Sudden severe sickness disrupts taken-for-grantedness. We tend to revisit the past to see if, after all, we might have predicted it.

Explanations for unexpected events are often called attributions by social psychologists. One group of researchers asked 30 parents, whose children had been diagnosed with cancer, the open-ended question: 'People sometimes say that they think about why their child became ill. Have you ever thought about this, and if you have, what sort of explanation have you come up with?' (Eiser et al., 1995: 33). Answers to these questions were found to divide into the following categories: none; genetic; environmental; unique trigger events; self-blame; and blame of spouse. A large percentage of mothers said that they blamed themselves. Parents were included in this category if they expressed concern about whether their smoking and dietary habits might have been significant. Another study examined 500 epidemiology questionnaires given to parents whose children were involved in treatment with Children's Cancer Group (CCG) protocols in the United States. At the end of the questionnaire concerning epidemiological factors that pertained to their children's cancer, parents were asked, 'Do you have any additional comments or concerns about anything that would have caused or contributed to you child's illness?' (Ruccione et al., 1994: 72). The majority of parents who responded to this question mentioned environmental factors that they thought might have contributed to their child's disease. The second most important concern was family health history. The other spontaneously mentioned causes and concerns were such things as chemicals in food, stress (either in a parent or a child), bewilderment, a sense of injustice, and geography (e.g., living near a polluting factory).

I, too, became interested in understanding more about childhood cancers. I wondered, how common are they? What are the causes thought to be? To answer these questions I turned to the epidemiological literature, which examines the incidence and prevalence (the number of new cases in a year and the number of cases in a population) of diseases along with the relationship between the incidence/prevalence and social, political, economic, and environmental factors. This field asks questions, for instance, about whether or not children living near nuclear power stations are more likely to be diagnosed with cancer.

In my search of the literature, I was happily surprised, on the one hand, to learn how very uncommon childhood cancer is. On the other hand, I was disturbed to see how the rates for childhood cancers are increasing. With respect specifically to leukemia, the rate among males 1-4 years of age in Canada was 7.5 per 100,000 in 1969-73 and 9.7 per 100,000 in 1993 , and, for females, 6.4 per 100,000 in 1969-73 and 7.3 per 100,000 in 1993 (Statistics Canada, 1997: 112). Clearly, this is a dramatic increase over the past 25 years, particularly for boys.

In numbers, there are about 910 children under 15 and 1,300 under 20 in Canada who develop cancer in a year (Desmeules, 1995: 1). Of these childhood cancers, the most common is leukemia. It accounts for about one-third of the new diagnoses and one-third of the deaths annually (Hutchcroft et al., 1996). Both the increasing incidence and the more positive prognoses have resulted in a situation where it is predicted that by the year 2000 one in every 900 young adults in North America (ages 16-34) will be a survivor of childhood cancer (Desmeules, 1995; 1). Generally, for most populations for which adequate data are available, the gender disparity ratios vary between 1.1 and 1.4 to 1, male to female. The incidence of leukemia is consistently higher among males than among females. Acute lymphoblastic leukemia is the most common form among children in most countries and reaches its highest rate among children under five. In a worldwide context, the incidence of childhood cancer varies a great deal, from 75 to 160 per million. In these terms its incidence in Canada is towards the high end, at 157 per million (see Table 1). Indeed, it is the most common cause of death among children 0-14 years of age (McBride, 1998).[3]

The search for the causes of childhood cancer takes us into the huge epidemiology research literature. There are thousands of studies from this perspective. They tend to examine correlations between rates of childhood cancers, or specific diagnostic categories of childhood cancer, and other things. For instance, there has been considerable research on various genetic, parental, occupational, and environmental conditions, including studies on diet, radiation, and electromagnetic rays and their relationship to a higher or lower incidence of various types of childhood cancer. Although there have been innumerable studies done in many countries looking at numerous possible causative factors and their relationships to different types of childhood cancer, there is still 'very little conclusive information' (ibid., 53). This is in part due to the many and difficult methodological issues faced by researchers in this field, including the lack of clarity about distinctions among different (etiologically) subtypes of disease, difficulties in accruing a significant number of cases for study, problems in measurement of environmental exposure levels, and lack of understanding of the biological mechanisms leading to childhood cancers (ibid.).

Children's cancers often differ from those of adults with respect to both their anatomy and the histology of the cell changes. Thus, the epidemiology of childhood cancer does not necessarily reflect

---

[3] I am shocked at these numbers. Although each week I would go to the clinic and see other patients, I never saw another of my own age. Because of this age discrepancy I felt very alone. Walking around my new university campus I felt the double isolation of newness and illness. Where were the others? Were there any others? It was not until I attended a young adult support group in the spring of 1997 in Toronto that I felt some release from the alienation of my disease. There I met others who 'knew', not just 'understood', what I was going through. That process was extremely therapeutic for me.

Table 1
Rates and Proportions of New Childhood Cancer Cases and Childhood Cancer Deaths in Canada

Cancer Type	New Cases		Deaths	
	Incidence Rate (1989–93)*	% of All New Cases	Mortality Rate (1991–5)*	% of All Cancer Death
Leukemia	48.1	30.7	9.39	32.2
Acute lymphocytic	38.3	24.4	4.22	14.5
Acute non-lymphocytic	6.0	3.8	2.22	7.6
Brain & Spinal	29.6	18.9	7.91	27.1
Astrocytoma	15.7	10.0	1.70	5.7
Medulloblastoma	5.2	3.3	1.76	6.0
Lymphoma	19.1	12.2	1.62	5.6
Hodgkin's disease	8.0	5.1	0.13	0.5
Non-Hodgkin's lymphoma	5.6	3.6	0.54	1.9
All other lymphomas	5.5	3.5	0.95	3.2
Sympathetic Nervous System	12.8	8.1	3.65	12.5
Soft Tissue	9.9	6.3	2.40	8.2
Renal Tumours	8.7	5.5	0.75	2.5
Carcinoma	7.5	4.8	0.47	1.6
Bone	7.2	4.6	1.58	5.4
Germ Cell	6.2	3.9	0.10	0.3
Retinoblastoma	3.7	2.4	0.03	0.1
Other Cancers	2.1	1.3	0.54	1.9
Hepatic Tumours	2.0	1.3	0.74	2.5
Total	156.8	100.0	29.19	100.0

*Rate per million children aged 0–14 years, standardized to the 1991 Canadian population.
SOURCE: National Cancer Institute of Canada, *Canadian Cancer Studies 1998* (Toronto, 1998). From McBride, 1998: 554.

that of adult cancers. This discussion will focus largely on childhood leukemia or ALL and will primarily use the findings of two review papers (Chow et al., 1996; McBride, 1998). First, a definition: leukemia essentially 'involves the proliferation of white cells in the blood which result from changes in the DNA of the stem cells from which white cells are manufactured in the bone marrow' and 'unrestrained production of immature lymphoblasts (a type of white cell) in the blood forming tissues, particularly the bone marrow, spleen, and lymph nodes' (Keene, 1997: 512).

A frequently studied cause of childhood leukemia is ionizing radiation exposure. The most dramatic empirical example of this is the increased incidence of leukemia among survivors and children of survivors of the atomic explosions at Hiroshima and Nagasaki near the end of World War II. Relatedly, more recently the rate of childhood thyroid cancer has increased dramatically in areas close to and most contaminated by the Chernobyl nuclear accident of 1986. The explosive increase in childhood thyroid cancer in Belarus, Ukraine, and the Russian Federation 'can be directly linked to the released radiation, and most likely to contamination by radioactive iodine isotopes' (Balter, 1995: 1758). While it is impossible to predict how many people will be affected, one estimate is that as many as one in 10 who were very young at the time of the accident and who were in the most heavily exposed areas could eventually be diagnosed with thyroid cancer. Moreover, 'we are seeing thyroid cancer 500 kilometres from Chernobyl. And in Europe everyone lives within 510 kilometres of a nuclear power station' (ibid., 1759).

Routine radiation *in utero* is another known cause of leukemia in children because of the heightened vulnerability of the fetus (see

Table 2
Mechanisms of Childhood Cancer Causation

Preconception maternal and paternal exposures:
- could result in transmissible genetic effects that could cause childhood cancer.

Prenatal maternal exposures:
- could result in in utero exposure of the developing infant to substances that cross the placental barrier and cause genetic or teratogenic effects, either directly to the mother or indirectly via transmission of exposures from other individuals in surroundings.

Postnatal maternal exposures:
- maternal exposures during the neonatal period, either direct or from other exposed individuals in surroundings, could result in transmission of exposures in breastmilk.

Postnatal exposure of child:
- child could be exposed directly or indirectly through others in surroundings.

SOURCE: Adapted from J. Peters and S. Preston-Martin, 'Childhood tumors and parental occupational exposures', *Teratogenesis, Carcinogenesis, and Mutagenesis* 4 (1984): 137–48. From McBride, 1998: 554.

Table 2). A number of studies using different research designs have been done. These enable researchers to make fairly reliable estimates. One such estimate is that the risk of cancer was increased by about 50 per cent, to those exposed in utero during a period between 1953 and 1967 when it was routine to X-ray pregnant women.

There is also evidence that children who live near high-tension electrical power lines and electrical substations have an increased likelihood of contracting leukemia. However, only a few studies and a very few children have been found to fall into this category. The available data, again, are problematic and thus the risk remains unknown. Moreover, although the research is not yet adequate for a clear finding of the implications of prenatal ultrasound for childhood leukemia, some research has suggested a link.

A viral infection of the mother during pregnancy has been investigated as potential cause of childhood leukemia. Even though it seems to be a weak risk factor because of its frequent occurrence in the population, its overall effect may be of some significance. Other infections, such as herpes and rubella, have been found in some studies to be associated with childhood cancer. There are also contradictory results with respect to postnatal exposure to viral infections. Some studies associate postnatal viral exposure with higher rates of leukemia, while others point to lower rates. Breast-feeding is found to be a protective factor in some studies but not in others. Clusters of leukemia have been observed in a number of different locations. While no specific infectious agents have been found, higher rates of leukemia among people in particular church or school groups have suggested the viability of a viral link.

Various drugs and chemicals have been investigated as possible correlates of childhood cancers. They become particularly potent threats when they are ingested by pregnant mothers because of the vulnerability of the fetus in utero. Although there is no consistent evidence linking maternal use of drugs, the following drugs have been studied to date with inconclusive results: anti-nausea medications, sedatives, sleeping pills, medications used for infections in pregnancy, and anti-convulsants. The effects on children of nitrosamine-containing substances such as burning incense, side-stream cigarette smoke, facial cosmetics, diuretics, anti-histamines, and cured meats and hot dogs have also been investigated inconclusively. As well, an association between maternal alcohol intake during pregnancy and childhood cancer has been examined without conclusive findings.

Other studies have looked at postnatal drug use. Contradictory and inconclusive results have been found with respect to the use of barbiturates, certain antibiotics, growth hormones, and even chemotherapy drugs used for a first cancer. Vitamins, particularly cod liver oil, which contains vitamins A and D, appear to have some protective effect for childhood leukemia. Various pesticides and insecticides have been found to have some association to childhood cancer, including leukemia.

Some hormones, such as DES (diethylstilbestrol), which was used in Canada between 1941 and 1970 to treat pregnant women at risk of miscarriage, have been associated with a rare form of cancer in young male and female offspring. The use of oral contraceptives within the three months prior to pregnancy has been related to an increased risk of leukemia. Some studies have found that babies whose mothers smoked during pregnancy have a much higher risk of various cancers. Other studies have related parental occupations to an increased incidence of childhood cancer. These include hydrocarbon-related work (gas station attendants, motor vehicle mechanics, and so on), work with chlorinated solvents (including paint sprays, dyes, or pigments), metal-related work, radiation-related employment, electromagnetic field exposure, and agriculture (because of pesticide exposure). Children whose mothers worked in pharmacies, bakeries, and factories and as physicians, pharmacists, or in pharmaceutical manufacturing or who were exposed to benzene, petroleum products, sawdust, soot, and organic dusts have been the subject of investigation. All of these factors have dubious association with childhood cancers.

A number of hereditary factors including ataxia-telangiectasia, Fanconi's anemia, neurofibromatosis, Li-Fraumeni syndrome, and Down's syndrome have a degree of association to childhood cancers. As well, there is some evidence of an increased risk associated with a family history of cancer. A number of birth characteristics, including increasing age of mother, being first-born, the mother's history of miscarriage and stillbirth, and elevated birth weight, have some relationships to childhood cancer in some studies.

Clearly, this review of the epidemiological literature provides a picture of how little is really known about the causes of childhood leukemia. It also demonstrates the shotgun and shot-in-the-dark approaches to research into the epidemiological causes of childhood cancer. It is no wonder, given the extremely variable approaches to the causes and the lack of unifying theory behind the myriad approaches, that so little is actually known. The various theories of causality are only part of the story of the lack of progress in this area. Another problem has to do with design issues. Generally speaking, there are a number of theories in medical/epidemiological research. The gold standard for medical research is thought to be the classic experimental design with 'before' and 'after' measures to at least two different groups, one of which receives the experimental condition (e.g., drug) while the other does not. Statistical comparisons depend on sample sizes that are large enough to be sensitive to a comparison of the measured difference between the experimental and control group. In this model human biology is thought to be a universal.

Epidemiological research, which focuses on the explanations for events based on their actual occurrence in the population, requires sample sizes that are large enough, and selected in such a way, to be representative of a population. In addition, the statistical analysis for epidemiological research design depends on the incidence of the hypothesized causal factors among the diseased population (e.g., children with ALL and pesticide use in the home). The less frequently either of these is found in the population the more difficult, in general, is proof of a correlation. Moreover, it is more difficult to control for competing causal links in population-based epidemiological studies. For instance, even if we find a strong correlation between childhood leukemia and pesticide use in the home we cannot be sure that pesticide use caused leukemia because the homes that used or didn't use pesticides and used various amounts of pesticides might also systematically vary in their parental smoking rates, degree of electromagnetic exposure, or even levels of hot dog consumption. Thus, the correlations found between pesticide use and leukemia may actually be the result of the correlation between hot dogs eaten in the home and leukemia.

The absence of an inclusive list of all the possible confounding variables and their control makes epidemiological research very difficult. It is also difficult because of such problems as geographic dispersion and population size. Knowledge that would lead to prevention seems, at first, to depend on such costly and logically and empirically difficult research.

The other type of research used in this field is animal research. In this case animals, most often mice or rats, are used as proxies for human beings. Then the factor that is hypothesized to cause the disease (e.g., pesticides for leukemia) is administered to the experimental mammal. If the mammal responds to pesticide ingestion by contracting leukemia there is evidence that the link should be the object of additional research. However, most cancers are thought to have a long latency period and thus take a long time to develop. This difficulty is addressed in part through the administration of exceedingly large amounts of the hypothesized causal substance to the (usually) small mammal. The amount of substance ingested (or applied) to shorten the latency period is usually many times larger than the amount that would be applied in a 'natural' setting. This is one of several factors that make the generalization from animals to humans problematic. (See Epstein, 1979, for a critical overview of the difficulties in using animals for cancer research.)

Social class, which encompasses such things as income and education, has repeatedly been shown to influence cancer incidence and mortality rates in a variety of adult cancers in the US and Canada. Very little research has been done on the impact of class on childhood cancer, although geographic location, which may at times be related to specific environmental exposure (e.g., radiation and pesticides), may also be related to social class. In one US study, the mortality rates for children with cancer whose parents received Aid to Families of Dependent Children were considerably and statistically significantly higher than for those whose parents were not receiving AFDC support (Nelson, 1992). Overall, from 28 days to 17 years of age, among White children, the mortality rate was in the order of 2.8 times greater for those receiving social assistance. Those of us in

Canada are able to think that this is largely or even entirely a function of the lack of universal health care. To some extent this may be the case. However, as the authors of the study note, this large class discrepancy 'points to the existence of social class differences in housing, nutrition, education, exposure to environmental risks', in addition to 'access to and use of health care and related services and facilities' (Nelson, 1992: 1133). Such differences exist in Canada and undoubtedly make a contribution to a differential mortality rate as well as to different degrees of suffering for children with cancer and their families. For instance, consider just the actual financial costs of driving to and parking at the hospital once per week for two years. At minimum the gas and parking costs would be $15. This figure ignores oil and 'wear and tear' on the automobile. Each trip for us took more than half a day and required us to miss two meals at home each time on average. Often, this would include two meals for three people. At minimum, this would be two meals for two people. A modest breakfast and lunch for two would be at least $20. Thus, even if a family were able to stick to these minimum expenses, which is unlikely, the annual out-of-pocket expense of weekly cancer therapy is nearly $2,000. In many cases one parent takes the time off work or will have to leave paid employment. I was fortunate in that I was eligible for a sabbatical in the year after Lauren's diagnosis. Still, the sabbatical required a 20 per cent loss in salary for one year.

A recent national Canadian study found that financial stress, even in a situation of universal health care, was second only to marital stress in causing problems for parents whose children had cancer. As the author indicates, this 'may be surprising because health care costs in Canada are almost exclusively covered by government programs, however, costs of lost wages, traveling to hospital or clinic, accommodation, meals, parking and babysitting are not covered.' In addition, 'financial difficulties were often encountered when one parent, usually the mother, was forced to cease employment, resulting in a marked reduction in family income' (Adams, 1992: 26). Clearly, class and income differentials in the impact of childhood cancer cannot be ignored.

My point in itemizing *just a few* of the costs is to suggest that financial penalties do exist, even with a universal health-care system.

Moreover, depending on the basic family income, these costs can be more or less crippling to the lifestyle of the whole family. The significance of such costs for the well-being of the ill child has not been empirically investigated. It needs to be. We know, for instance, that social support is of benefit to quality of life and longevity for women with breast cancer (Spiegal, 1991), and in numerous other studies support is associated with positive health outcomes (see Lerner, 1994, for a balanced overview of the findings about the association between social psychological issues such as social support and health outcomes).

Two competing conclusions can be drawn. On the one hand, we could argue that more research needs to be done to understand the social class and environmental correlates of childhood cancer. On the other hand, there are those who argue that we do not know conclusively about the specific causes of childhood cancer and, furthermore, because of the exceedingly high levels of proof required by science, it is unlikely that this will be accomplished in the near future. After all it took more than a half-century between the time that findings demonstrated a link between smoking and lung cancer and the discovery of conclusive, genetic change. In addition, environmental activists argue, there are a sufficient number of consistent patterns of correlation between various types of cancers and numerous chemicals already unregulated and used extensively in the environment (Colburn et al., 1996; Steingraber, 1997; Epstein, 1998). Instead of allowing the continued use of chemicals, as well as radon and other products associated with nuclear power, until absolute scientific proof is available it is critical that precautions be taken. Substances repeatedly found to be carcinogenic in animal, mapping, and residue studies should be banned and taken off the market and replaced with substances that are harmless. There are already legislative moves in this direction.

Meta-analysis of the studies that have been done needs to be pursued. Unifying and distinguishing theories that would find the commonalities and the uniqueness of environmental and social class explanations need to be developed. Stopping the growing rate and preventing this disease are urgent.

According to McBride (1998: S53) there is reason for optimism:

In recent years, [with] rising new classifications of childhood cancers and improved methodologies in large collaborative epidemiologic studies, more confirmation is available on the potential factors affecting the risk of childhood cancers. Much further research is required, however, since in many areas of study, specific agents have not been conclusively identified, mechanisms of carcinogenesis have not been determined, and exposure assessment that could provide information on relevant timing, quantity, and modes of exposure is lacking.

Chapter 4

Remission Induction: Boot Camp in Hospital Living

'We kill all the cells with "methotrexate" over the first few days, then send in "citrovorum" to save the good ones.' This is the way that remission induction was described to us. It was to happen on a Friday, the day after the announcement of the diagnosis. The first step was to move Lauren (and me) to another room—one with 'negative' pressure. This was one of five rooms along the back of the ward, all designed for treatment when a child was neutropenic, i.e., didn't have enough neutrophils, a type of white cells, in his or her blood to fight off an infection. This room was in the corner and it had a bathroom of its own. It was, as all the negative-pressure rooms are, a large single room with a couch for a sleeping parent. The idea of 'killing all the cells' was science fiction/horror to me at the time. The fear that they wouldn't really be able to save the good cells lurked in the far reaches of my mind.[1] Looking back, I can hardly believe that we didn't stop the action here. But what choice did we have—we didn't even really think of a second opinion. We had talked briefly about it, but we were convinced by the kindness of the doctor and his optimism. We were still in a land of shock.

After all, this was a teaching hospital with a very good reputa-

---

[1] Although I remember little from this time, one instance of the initial chemotherapy injection stays with me. It was late at night, 2 a.m. or so, and a nurse entered. She was not wearing the usual teddy-bear top and blue pants that seem to be a favourite of pediatric nurses. Instead, she was fully gowned, gloved, hairnetted, and masked. She was glowing, for the yellow-green of the gown reflected the flashing of the intravenous machine. In her hand she carried a large sac filled with what seemed to be pulsing orange fluid. It had a large skull-and-crossbones sticker plastered on its front. Without any explanation, she attached this to my machine, sending this poisonous fluid into my body. What was I to think! How could positive visualization change this image? How could the skull and crossbones become little daisies floating in my blood? This was a very traumatic experience for me, caused by her attire and lack of explanation of her purpose.

tion. And I guess we didn't want to wait. Somehow, we accepted unknowingly, and relatively unthinkingly, the urgency of beginning treatment. Those days of remission induction—those 30 days—are a blur now. I didn't eat and only drank coffee. Lauren felt sick, tired, out of sorts. When we entered she had felt fine, except for the dizziness and headaches when she climbed stairs or stood up quickly. A new 'miracle' drug, ondonstetron, was injected intravenously and was supposed to be amazing. As they gave it to her, the nurses told Lauren how wonderful this drug was and how much difference it made. As recently, I gathered, as five years earlier, remission induction had involved almost constant nausea and vomiting. She felt nauseated and her tummy felt sore, but she didn't vomit very often or very much. Her body did not, however, behave the way it normally did. She slept and half-slept most of the time. Later, Cindy said that she remembered this as a time when Lauren hovered between living and dying. I didn't at the time, however, realize how tenuous her hold on life was. I was buoyed up by the optimism in the doctor's diagnosis and by my need to help Lauren feel as comfortable as possible. At this time, too, Jess, Richard, and Marian were coming down each morning and staying for the day. Visitors were coming each evening. And medical staff of various sorts were coming and going.

The land of shock is an unfamiliar one. I am surprised at myself and my reaction to Lauren's diagnosis and the events that followed. Now, four years later, I ask myself, why weren't we or why wasn't I sceptical? I, as a person trained in the ironic detachment of the sociologist to boot, am particularly surprised by what looks from the distance of a few years to be naïvety because of our open trust of this one particular doctor, in this one particular place. I had learned so much about medical error and about how personal, financial, familial, sociodemographic (race, class, and gender), and other interests affect what doctors determine to be the best possible treatments at any one point in time (Clark et al., 1991) that I look in surprise at my almost totally uncritical response in this case. To use a contemporary and popular expression, I didn't have 'a clue'. I had only thought of cancer in others—women with breast cancer, children several generations ago. I had never thought of it as a part of my story—well, maybe yes, but when I am much, much,

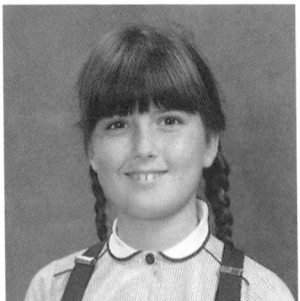

Lauren at five, 1983.

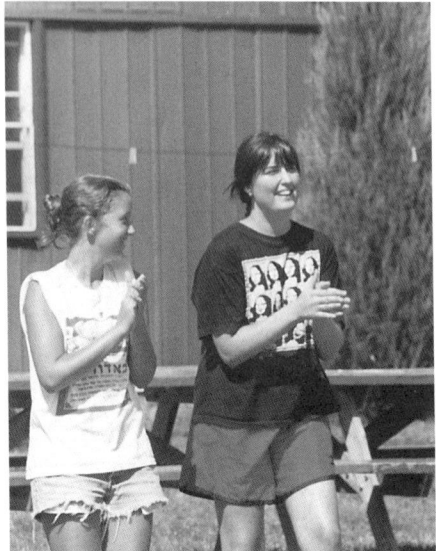

Lauren just before the diagnosis in August at a retreat for the high school student council, August 1995.

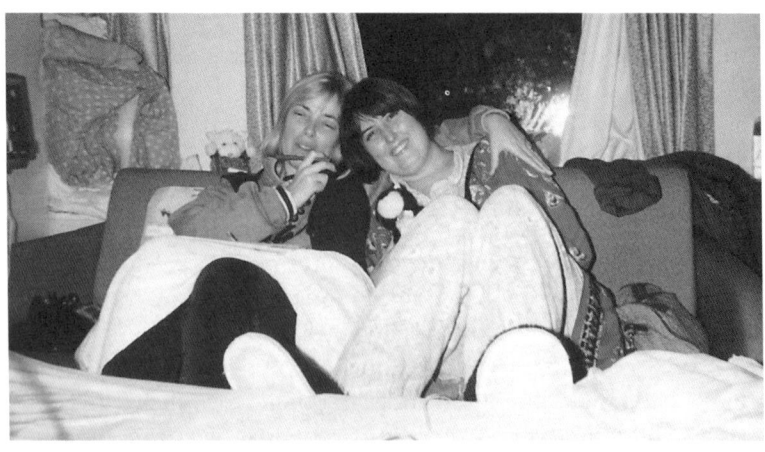

Juanne and Lauren in the hospital during remission induction, October 1995.

Remission Induction: Boot Camp in Hospital Living 🙶 49

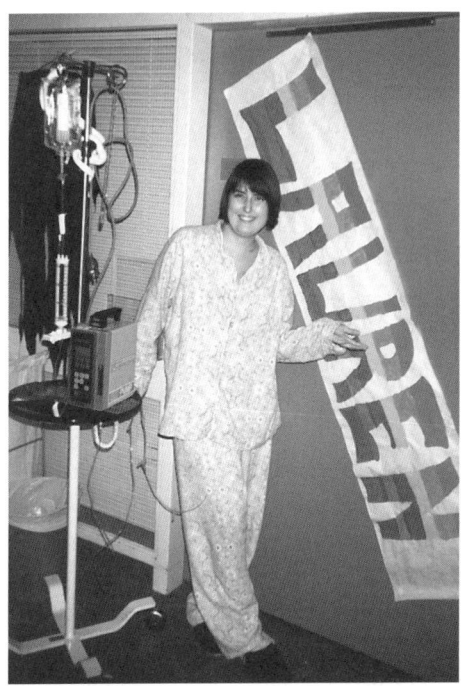

The sign on Lauren's hospital room door, about two and a half weeks into the remission induction stage of treatment, October 1995.

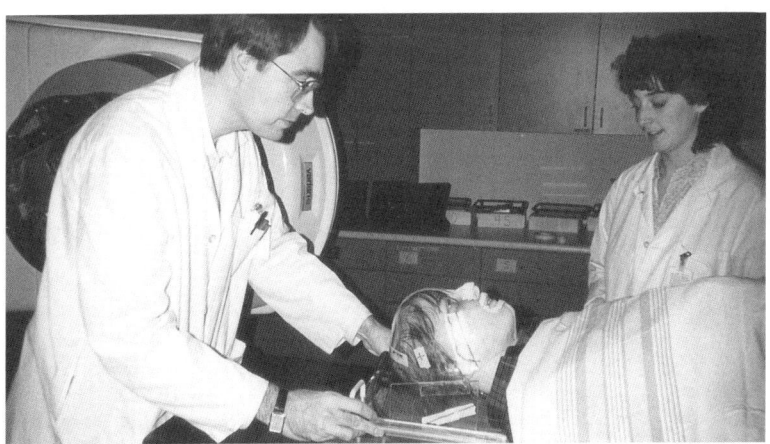

Lauren preparing to begin radiation.

much older. Never as a story of the life of one of my children. Nevertheless . . .

Marian, Lauren's dad, and Jess went home to Kitchener-Waterloo each night and each day brought back more and more stuff to make Lauren's stay as comfortable as possible. When Lauren had run for school council president the previous spring, her best friend had made a fabulous rainbow poster representation of her name. It became the decoration for her door. Marian bought new warm slippers for Lauren and a wonderful whiteboard for the wall. Richard and Marian also brought their portable stereo with CDs. We used the whiteboard to list the names of the nurses, visitors, and meals for the day. Each day Lauren wrote on this and decorated it with coloured markers.[2] Flowers and cards started to arrive. Lauren asked for and received a number of posters from her bedroom walls. These we placed on the walls of her hospital room. Her French homeroom class made a huge multi-page sign that included pictures of all the kids, individual by individual, manipulating their bodies in various alphabetical shapes to spell out their greetings and good wishes. Within a few days the room was hers. Balloons, posters, flowers, cards, and notes were everywhere.[3]

Jess stayed over with her dad and Marian the first weekend, from the diagnosis on Thursday to the following Sunday night, then called a couple of friends to come to the hospital to meet her and go back with her to her apartment. None of us could face having Jess return alone to her home on public transport after such a momentous event. Each week after that, Jess stayed at school, Monday to Wednesday, and then arrived at the hospital on Wednesday night to spend the rest of her time with her sister. We talked, slept, watched videos, listened to music. We ended the day by focusing on what positive there had been in what was other-

---

[2] It was a good day if I could write on this blackboard. I remember many days when I didn't have the energy and it was others (Marian, mostly) who wrote and decorated the board. This blackboard was a cheerful help to me. It listed all the positive things in my day and gave a sense of continuity and routine.

[3] My room was literally both a flower and card shop after the first week. Dozens of roses, carnations, birds of paradise sat in vases, and 'Peanuts' and 'Far Side' cards covered my wall. It was as cheerful as a medical room could be.

wise a terrible situation and tried to write about three good things that happened each day.[4]

After a few days, Lauren started to feel better and Marian and Richard brought down my new laptop computer. Lauren started to write a magazine for teenagers with cancer, which she later handed in for a creative writing workshop, a part of one of her courses. She had been in the middle of applying for scholarships, and she and I had been working on her résumé. Come to think of it, I had been doing the mechanical work—hand-printing her mailing address and the other information that had to be done but that did not take thinking, because she was so tired and busy. She was not able to finish filling in her scholarship applications and she didn't even know whether she'd get back to school to finish her year. She didn't know whether to take two years or one year to finish her OACs (final, optional year of high school in Ontario, a year of college prep courses). She applied to university, just in case that was what she wanted to do. So that she would not be 'just another patient' she gave a copy of her résumé to the doctors and nurses for 'her' chart. Dr Q read this and noted that his daughter had been at the same debating championships in Ottawa the previous spring. The conversation in which he talked about his daughter and Lauren and debating cemented our trust, respect, and care for Dr Q.

During these times, too, a number of other hospital personnel visited—the two nutritionists, two different pharmacists, the teacher, the social worker, the woman who was to be Lauren's nurse from the clinic—a veritable merry-go-round of residents, doctors, and others. One after another, these various professionals knocked and entered our room. We never knew what we had in store for us. As each new professional arrived, a new personal style and new information were bestowed on us as well. One nutrition-

---

4 Our goal was three things. Often this list expanded. Sometimes we filled pages of notes with what people had said or done, what food I'd enjoyed, who had called, etc. I also remember a few days when this list was not possible to do, and the end result of discussion was tears of frustration. However, usually we could find some humorous notation to include that would lighten the mood and ease my sleep. I look back now and wonder how we could have seen so much good in so much pain. My dad often provided funny and positive incidents for the board.

ist/dietitian, a true pessimist, told us about her brother-in-law's impending death and about the girl who had just relapsed after two years of treatment with the same disease that Lauren had. She rose above her gloomy outlook to be impressed with Lauren's diet. She asked her what an average day's menu prior to diagnosis was. She gave Lauren questionnaires to fill out about her dietary likes and dislikes. Lauren had mentioned that she liked Perrier water and yoghurt with live culture. Every day thereafter, there was a brown paper bag labelled for Lauren in the fridge with a bottle of Perrier, yoghurt, and a piece of fresh fruit. She was put on a vegetarian diet and told she could order doubles whenever she wanted. Though pessimistic and sad, we enjoyed her visits—she was accessible and real as a person, and told stories of her family, her job, her job prospects. We felt like reaching out to her to offer support in her struggles.[5]

Then there was a pharmacist who sat beside Lauren as she lay half-awake, half-asleep with intravenous drugs dripping into her and, in a monotone, recited the interminable list of all the side-effects of all the drugs that Lauren would be taking in the next two years. She didn't ask if Lauren wanted to know, if Lauren understood, if Lauren wanted her to go slower, to write anything down—nothing like that. She simply carried on. She seemed to have the information memorized and flawlessly recited it, without feeling, and without allowing us any time to understand what it was she was saying.

We did not think there was a choice of drugs, in any case. This was a very serious disease and the treatment protocol Lauren was on, we had been told, had proven to be successful in the treatment of the disease. Side-effects or late-effects were irrelevant to us at this time. Stopping the disease process that had been going on in her body was primary. We had already decided to go ahead. This list just added worries. We had decided that Lauren would go through

---

5   This nutritionist offered my mom and me some comic relief in the hospital. Whenever she would enter we would be the ones helping her, not the opposite. We really were supportive. After she left we would shake our heads at this. She was very nice, however, and helpful in regard to nutrition.

> **A Note to Nurses and Doctors**
>
> As a teen patient of leukemia I am in a unique position. I am curious and can understand the issues of my illness. When you speak of my blood counts, my bodily functions, my procedures I can comprehend what is being said. I feel that I am more fortunate than a younger child because I know that what you are doing is not trying to hurt me, but heal and cure me. The one unfortunate side-effect of my being able to understand is that I sometimes hear things that I don't need to know. I want to know what treatment is coming up. I want to know about my protocol. However, I feel that I have also been told things I do not need to know. First, I'd like to speak about pain. In particular, I do not need to know about the pain involved in an operation or procedure months before the procedure takes place. I do not need to worry far in advance. I do not need to worry about the 'next' pain before I am through the current one. For me, the level of pain I can expect can be left until the day before. That would be helpful. The second issue is that of side-effects. With leukemia every single person reacts differently to every drug, radiation, and procedure. In general, I find it disturbing to hear lists of side effects. Although I do want to know the side-effects so that I can be prepared and not completely afraid when something occurs, oral lists do not work for me. Each side-effect that comes out of your mouth is truly like a jolt to my psyche. Perhaps a handwritten list would be better. In this way I can browse through it, when I am emotionally up to it. In general, you tell me what I need and want to know. I appreciate that and wish that to continue. But as a teen patient, and I hope I can speak on behalf of at least a few others, I can understand and therefore need to be treated more gently. Thank-you very much.
>
> From Lauren's magazine for teen cancer patients, *Healing Hands, Fighting Fists* (Spring 1996).

with the treatment, and so this was terrifying information. It is, however, required by law, and so we all had to go through the motions. Come to think of it, the timing of this was a bit odd. Permission for treatment was actually to have been preceded by the information as to side-effects and long-term effects. But this happened after treatment had started. The urgency of beginning the treatment had apparently superseded the ethics protocol.

The principle of informed consent is supposed to include much more than we were ever told and should have been concluded before Lauren ever started treatment.

> Informed consent requires that (1) all the treatments available to the child have been laid on the table and discussed—not just the treatment available at your hospital or through your doctor, but all the treatments that could be beneficial, wherever they are given; (2) the parents and, to the extent possible, the child, have discussed these options and decided that they want to consider one of them; (3) the option selected is thoroughly discussed, with all its benefits and risks clearly explained. A fully informed medical decision weighs the relative merits of a therapy after full disclosure of benefits, risks, and alternatives. (Keene, 1997: 76)

Clearly, this was not the ethics protocol we received.

The pharmacist seemed to be in a hurry to get it all out—almost in one gulp. I guess she had gone through this list many times. We were being drowned by the newness of lost hair, liver, pancreatic, spleen, and kidney damage, heart failure, paralysis, weakness, fatigue, bone marrow depression, mouth sores, tingling hands and feet, muscle atrophy, bone pain, and so on. Finally and abruptly, I interrupted her and said, 'You'll have to go now; we've had enough.' At least she listened and left.

The next time we had a question we asked the other pharmacist to come to the room to provide the answer. The steroid that Lauren was taking gave her waking nightmares.[6] She was talking in

---

6 These nightmares were the most graphic I've ever had. They were in brilliant colours, with loud sounds and lots of action. They kept me feeling awake all the time. I had a recurring dream that made me feel as though I could never awake from it. This dream was filled with streams of blood that I tried to ride out on a raft, yet never quite succeeded. All of my nightmares contained lots of blood, everywhere. I remember this blood being in pools, or shadows, and dripping, dripping. I was very glad when they stopped, due to a medication change a few weeks after we left the hospital.

her sleep and not feeling rested in the morning. We wondered if these symptoms were typical, were related to the steroid, and could be alleviated in some way. By this time one more drug seemed an easy and benign solution. We had become so quickly used to reliance on pharmaceuticals! We, who had seldom even had Tylenol in our home. We, who had relied on vitamin C, echinacea, honey and lemon, rest, and pleasure for good health! He said that, yes, perhaps they could give Lauren something else to eliminate or minimize the side-effects if they continued after she was out of the hospital. He left stiffly—perhaps thankful to be finished with these people who questioned the treatment and who had asked his colleague to leave.

The social worker arrived one day, pamphlets from the Candlelighters Foundation, the Ronald McDonald House, and Camp Trillium in hand to give to us. This seemed to be all she had time for. We were delighted when the chaplain was to come, but she, too, could only stay for a short time.

The teacher, on the other hand, was a breath of fresh air. She represented Lauren's chance for a return to normality—a return to her former self and what she had been doing before. She said that she could contact Lauren's school and make arrangements to get course work and negotiate about Lauren's course requirements for the rest of the semester. As Lauren was taking a film studies course, she offered to get Lauren some of her course films to watch in the hospital room. And she did. Those not available at the public library she borrowed from her son-in-law's collection. A virtual Academy Award bonanza of classic and modern films—esoteric and mundane, profound and profane—arrived in the days remaining in the hospital. The teacher was always helpful. She was direct. She had a specific service to offer Lauren and it was valuable.[7]

Perhaps the most astonishing of this panoply of 'professional' visitors was the radiation resident. He came into Lauren's isolation room, coughing and clearing his throat. Now it's hard to know what

---

7 Again, as with any of the really 'good' practitioners I met, the teacher saw me as a real person and not solely as a body to be fixed. I was just the same as any other student, but I needed a little extra arranging to get back to the required learning. She was easy, fun, and supportive of me.

to do in a situation like this. He was a doctor, for heaven's sake. He had been around these wards of sickness, cancer, and radiation for years. We had been in the ward for less than 10 days. He'd know, wouldn't he, if he had a cold and shouldn't come in? Maybe it was nervous mannerism, maybe just a genetic anomaly, one that didn't involve germs, just throat noises. Okay, I said to myself, he must know what he is doing.

He explained his purpose. Lauren was to have 10 days of cranial radiation. As is the legal standard of care today, she had to be informed ahead of time of the potential side-effects (although, as indicated above, she heard this list and the list of the effects of the chemotherapy after it had started, not before) and had to sign a form agreeing that, in spite of the dangers, she was willing to undergo the risk. The radiology resident, as the pharmacist had previously done, listed the risks in a monotone—they must all go to the same drama school—but when he came to reporting on a study in which the average loss of intellectual functioning from radiation to the head was 10 IQ points, I had, once again, to ask the health-'care' provider to leave Lauren's room. 'Please leave right now', I said. 'This is not acceptable.'

He had been reporting on one recent study. I have since learned that there are numerous studies documenting various cognitive impairments after cranial radiation. One study was being used as a flagship. The average age of youngsters with leukemia in this study was four. The average age of most children in all studies would have to be much lower than Lauren's 17 because the mean age for a leukemia diagnosis was four. Lauren's brain was at a different stage of development. The findings could not be generalized, could they? He had to leave! Besides, whether there was any truth or not, having decided to save her life, information about the side-effects of what we believed to be necessary treatment was not only too late, it was secondary. However, had this information been coupled with short-, medium-, and long-term strategies to alleviate possible problems based on educational theory or what I know to have been decades of research on the relative malleability of the brain and the potential to 'regain lost cells', it might have been of help.

This assault was probably the worst (at the time) to Lauren.

Losing IQ points signified losing herself. Lauren started to cry. I went out to the nursing station and said I urgently needed to talk to another 'expert'. I explained what had happened. One of the nurses came in and hugged Lauren. The radiation oncology nurse, a woman with great savoir faire, came by quickly and explained that the resident had been wrong to say what he did. She emphasized the positive—the perfectionism of the doctor in charge of the radiation, the relatively low level of dosage, the fact that there were likely very few side-effects.[8]

Within the next few days, everyone, it seems, had heard the tale of this 'atrocity'. We had hit a nerve in our complaints about the resident. Then doctors, residents, and nurses came by to apologize and to say that what he had done/said had been wrong. He was apparently 'spoken to' by the doctor in charge of radiation. I still don't know how much of the problem was due to cultural differences: he seemed to have a slight accent and appeared to be of an ethnic minority. The 'facts' he was describing were true—i.e., he was reporting on the results of at least one recent study of the long-term effects of radiation to the heads of children with leukemia. The problem was that he didn't couch the study results in qualifications and limitations and didn't emphasize the characteristics of the study sample, such as younger age and developing brains, educational background, and so on. But then, the resulting reaction of his colleagues almost seemed an overreaction to me, not because he was right to do what he did, after all, but because it seemed to me something that might best have been dealt with privately, between him and his supervisor. Instead, because of the 'team' care approach, it seemed that everyone knew and pronounced judgement.

These days in the hospital passed both slowly and quickly. Time changes its meaning in the hospital. It flies by. Then it hobbles. The markers of time on the outside—sunrise and sunset, school and work beginning and ending, lunch and break hours—

---

8   The hug of my nurse and the subsequent rational explanation by the radiation nurse helped me immeasurably. Again, I was being seen as a person. People also started joking that I could afford to lose a few IQ points, and this was a reassuring stroke to my damaged ego.

provide time with a recognizable structure. Most of these markers, these distinctions, are obliterated in hospitals. Hospitals are busy all night long and all day long. Many nights we woke to the smell and the sound of popcorn popping in the microwave oven, after midnight for the nightshift break for the nurses on duty. Even though lights were out after midnight, temperature-taking and pill-taking continued. Day and night were constantly being interrupted by one or another of the health-care team.

There were other problems. Lauren was in an isolation room. Outside her door was a sink for washing hands. Everyone, including the nursing staff, was supposed to wash before entering her room. All of Lauren's private visitors did. I did. Her sister did. Her father and stepmother did. My sister did. In fact, Cindy had even explained that we were to wash up to our elbows. Little rules such as hand-washing became immensely important. We were fixated. This was

---

Hospital Smile

It was very dark, the only light was an eerie red from the intravenous machine. Flashing, flashing, incessantly.

Then the door opened. A flurry of activity commenced. Pulse taken. Temperature checked.

Still vital? The patient was.

And then a quiet 'Lauren?'

'Yes?'

'It's Theresa.' The nurse told her sleepy patient.

'Hi. What time is it?'

'Oh, two a.m.' I brought you some lemon drops. You can give them out to nurses with bad breath if you want!' She laughed out loud.

'Thank-you.' The patient smiled and rolled over to sleep again.

Hospital time again . . . The patient was awake, so why not give her lemon drops at two a.m.?

Why not indeed!

From Lauren's magazine for teen cancer patients, *Healing Hands, Fighting Fists* (Spring 1996).

one thing that we could do to help prevent the development of any more problems in a situation where we lacked both control itself and any sense of control, and where we lacked even basic knowledge. Following the rules became rigidly and ritualistically important for us. Although the doctors were generally overheard washing their hands, it seemed, as we listened, that almost no other healthcare professional did. As well, to heighten our anxiety there was the continuous entrance and exit of doctors, residents, nurses, interns, medical students, cleaners, porters, even, one day, two high school students who wanted to be doctors. Lauren's rest was certainly compromised. Undoubtedly, germs were multiplied.

One night, one of the nurses outside was coughing and sneezing and blowing her nose. Earlier she had come into Lauren's room and changed her intravenous medications. Later, when I heard her coughing, I went outside to the nurses' desk to check who was coughing and blowing her nose. When I saw that it was the nurse who had just been into Lauren's room, I asked her not to come back. She obviously had a bad cold. Shortly after, this same nurse came back into the room to check again on the equipment and medications. I had to get up and ask her again to leave and to stay out. I then went to tell the other nurse on duty what I had requested/demanded. This 'coughing' nurse stayed out of our room the rest of that night, but I have no doubt that she nursed in other critical-care isolation rooms. I spoke to her supervisor as soon as I could. The supervisor must have talked with this nurse because about three days later she tearfully apologized to me. She said she wouldn't hurt any of the kids 'for anything'. I said I believed her and forgave her. We hugged and that was that.

A few days later another nurse, this time one with a cold sore on her mouth, was working at the isolation room end of the floor. We had been warned about the dangers of chicken pox and the related herpes virus for people on chemotherapy, so I was upset and concerned. Early in the treatment we had been given a package of materials about the treatment protocol. On a list entitled 'When to Contact the Clinic', the first item was, 'your child has been exposed to or develops chickenpox, or another infection'. Again, I had to speak to a supervisor. This time the nurse in question was

> **To My Nurses**
> I am afraid of my illness
> I am afraid of the pain
> I am afraid of all the
> unknowns
> But sometimes
> I am afraid of you
> Because you see ...
> I can hear you talking about
> taking my blood and giving
> me finger pokes in the hall
> I can see that you are sometimes eating when you
> change my IV bags
> I can hear that you don't always wash your hands
> before you come into my
> room
> And at times I hear you
> coughing and sniffling
> outside.
> You see ...
> I can see
> I can hear
> And I can be afraid
>
> From Lauren's magazine for teen cancer patients, *Healing Hands, Fighting Fists* (Spring 1996).

sent to 'infection control' and was told that she was no longer contagious. We had to accept that. She continued nursing at the other end of the isolation ward but we didn't see her again.[9]

Hospitals aren't necessarily the cleanest or most sanitary

---

9   I can still feel my fear at seeing the cold sore and hearing the coughing. You see, there I was, isolated, afraid, already lying in my bed trying to stay healthy, fighting for my life. In walks a nurse who looks like she could (and might) cause me to die! Although it may sound like an overreaction, that is what I felt. I did not need any other possible illnesses.

places to be. One night I got up to go to the bathroom and walked down the hall only to see a mouse. I went to the nursing station to report this, thinking, of course, that someone would deal rapidly with such a shocking intrusion into a pediatric oncology ward filled with children with life-threatening illnesses. The fellow behind the desk working at the computer said, when I had reported what I had seen, 'Oh yes, we have mice and rats here.' I couldn't believe his response and so I went to the parents' lounge and phoned the pediatric oncologist on call, who explained, 'We have to fumigate every six months or so; there are problems with the building and mice get in.' And this was thought to be one of the best hospital/medical schools in Canada at the time.

I engaged a few nurses in conversation about these occurrences and learned that many of the nurses didn't feel they could refuse an offer to work—sick or not—because of the terrible stress and tension they were under as hospitals, wards, and beds closed throughout Ontario in the mid-nineties. Sick nurses at work were a sign of the times. Many were only part-time and they could not refuse work without losing money (sick leave was not a part of their contracts). They needed the money to feed and house their children and they were insecure because so many of their friends and colleagues were losing jobs. So they hoped for the best for their patients and hoped no parents noticed or complained (the way I did) so that they could make a living for themselves and their families.

How did I spend my time when Lauren was sleeping, doing homework, or reading? Doing nothing. I sat or lay down on the couch beside her bed. I couldn't think. I couldn't read. I couldn't eat. I couldn't talk on the phone. For the most part I simply tried to calm myself with meditation and prayer. Hours and hours and hours. I had work to do. I had publication deadlines. I had friends and family who cared. But I was unable to do anything except deal with immediate issues related to Lauren's care and sit empty-minded.

There is an intensity to all of life that accompanies serious and life-threatening illness. Broyard (1992) called this the 'intoxication of illness'. Everything once taken for granted is opened to question and examination. One looks more closely at all that is around. My tasks had changed radically. I was host to doctors, residents, interns, nurses, cleaning persons, kitchen servers, teachers, pharmacists, social workers, chaplains, and others.[10] During the day and evenings, I hosted parents of intimate friends of Lauren's, teachers from Lauren's school. Guarding Lauren against unkindness; helping and comforting her when she felt sick; walking her to the washroom day and night with her IV pole; calling nurses to measure urine 'output' before they 'dumped her hat' (a container that fits over the toilet to capture urine), the output of which must be measured; changing Lauren's bedclothes and linens and finding new ones on the ward in the middle of the night when she had a 'night sweat'; juggling telephone calls—these were the activities of which my days and nights were made.

She was sick to her stomach once in a while. Almost nightly she sweated so that her pyjamas and bedding were soaking wet. In the first few days she mostly just slept, worked on her laptop computer, vomited, and rose to go to the bathroom periodically. After the first few days, when the drug designed to save the good cells was administered, she started to feel more energetic and asked periodically about when she could leave the hospital.

Once Lauren was through the remission induction and her blood counts, particularly the neutrophil counts, had started to go up, she was allowed to go home. We had been anxiously awaiting this day, which was about two weeks after the diagnosis and the beginning of treatment. On the way home, though, Lauren had to have a second fitting for a mask for her cranial irradiation so that the beams could be directed at a narrowly specified, demarcated part of her head. There are several fittings of the mask, which is made precisely for the individual patient so that it protects the part of the cranium not being irradiated. The first time we had gone for a fitting it had been in an ambulance travelling from one hospital to another. Lauren was feeling really ill at the time and yet had to

---

10 My mom has an amazing ability to put others at ease, whether they are waitpersons or friends, colleagues or doctors. She was always hospitable and kind to the nurses (unless they did something wrong). She would ask them how they were doing and sympathize with their situations. All of this was done sincerely, with the wondrous side-effect that I believe we got better treatment than would have otherwise been the case. People responded positively to my mom most of the time.

lie flat on a stretcher while she was pushed through the halls to the downstairs door where ambulances dropped off and picked up their fares. She also had to lie flat on the stretcher as the ambulance bumped across busy city streets torn up by construction. I was afraid she was going to vomit and that we would be unable to keep her at all comfortable. Not only, though, was the ride an excruciating exercise in 'holding on', but Lauren had to stay absolutely still on her back while she was fitted for the radiation mask. The people doing the fitting were really friendly and kind. They had a blanket warmer and brought a warm blanket over while we waited and then gave Lauren a new warmed blanket while she was being fitted. At times like these, a warm blanket was heavenly! These small, kindly touches were so appreciated.[11]

When she was finished with the fitting Lauren seemed to my hand (putting my hand on her forehead became a routine for me over the next two years or so) to have an elevated temperature and so before we left the hospital to drive the hour or so home I asked a nurse to take her temperature so that we would know that she was okay. She was. It was normal and so we set off. Lauren was too weak to walk to the car through the lobby to the elevator and so had to ride in a wheelchair and then be helped into the car. Marian drove and I sat in the back with Lauren's head on my lap. When we arrived home I got out of the car and opened the front door of the house, then went back to the car. Marian and I helped Lauren into the house. A friend of Lauren's walked by and said, 'Hi, you don't look as bad as I thought you would.'[12] By the time we reached our

---

11 For many reasons I was glad to be a pediatric patient. One was that I feel I got more personal care from the nurses, though I do not know this for certain. Another is that the chemotherapy doses are stronger for children than adults because their bodies can handle them better. This means they worked harder at saving me. Finally, a radiation attendant told me, to waylay my fears, that the radiation was so directed that it was within millimetres of the correct location. On the other hand, if I were an adult it would have only been within centimetres, which is still relatively safe. The theory is that a child still has 60, 70, even 80 years to live, while an adult has fewer years. Therefore, my future quality of life, as a pediatric patient, was more protected than it would have been if I had been diagnosed five months later as an 'adult'.

12 This incident was at the time horrid and hysterically funny. The friend was someone I had known since the time I was 10 years old. His forte had never been sensitivity. However, he did make the brave effort to come to see me, and for this I am thankful.

family room Lauren was shivering, her teeth were chattering, and she said she was freezing. I ran upstairs and got a bunch of blankets, brought them down, and wrapped her in them. I lay beside her on the couch trying to keep her warm. But her forehead was hot. What a confusing situation! We decided to take her temperature.

We had one thermometer, the one I had bought that day long ago (two weeks, in fact) at the urgent-care clinic when the doctor on duty had said that if her temperature went above 38.5 degrees Celsius I was to take her to the hospital. This time her temperature was elevated—over 40 degrees Celsius. I couldn't believe it. I didn't understand. How could she be shivering so, feeling internally cold, with such a high fever? We went to the neighbours' house to borrow another thermometer. By this time her dad had arrived on his way home from work. No one was home at the neighbours, so Richard drove quickly to the nearest drugstore for another thermometer. Meanwhile, we took her temperature again. It was now normal. Whew! But she still felt cold. She was still shivering. How could her temperature be varying so much? There must be something wrong with the thermometer.

I called the hospital. By the time I got through to the nurse, Richard had come back and we had taken Lauren's temperature with the new thermometer. Again it registered above 40 degrees. They could not both be right, I thought. Her temperature at one moment was over 40 and at the next 38 degrees. I was still trying to keep Lauren cosy. The nurse said that Lauren was febrile and that we had to bring her back to the hospital immediately. They had warned us that in the case of an elevated temperature, whenever Lauren was neutropenic, we had to be at the hospital within an hour. All four of us instantly got organized for this emergency drive back to the hospital, which normally took an hour. Richard drove his car. Marian sat in the front seat and Lauren and I resumed our back-seat locations— Lauren as flat out as possible with her head on my lap. This was one of the scariest times for all of us. Lauren said she loved us.[13] Later on

---

13 This was the one time that I thought the end had come. My temperature kept varying and I felt very sick. I had it in my head that if my temperature got past a certain point I would lose my sense of reason. I wanted my family to know that I loved them in case I could not tell them this the next morning.

she said that she thought she was going to die. We stopped for bottled water on the way down the highway and I tried to get Lauren to drink as much as possible, with a straw, to keep her temperature down. She drank and drank—as much as she could.[14]

We arrived at the emergency ward and were placed in a private alcove with curtains and began a wait for the doctor. Finally, several hours later, she was readmitted. The next day one of the doctors said Lauren should not have been sent home because her 'counts' were so low and this febrile reaction was predictable. The other doctor had agreed to let her go home on the belief, he said, that if she got into trouble (e.g., experienced a raised temperature) we would bring her back, and in the meantime she would likely be happier at home. Nevertheless, both when she was initially diagnosed and just after she had been allowed home after her remission induction, we arrived within the hour at the hospital only to wait for hours and hours in the emergency department for a doctor to admit Lauren.

Lauren was admitted this time for another course of antibiotics and until her neutrophil counts returned to normal.[15] This was still within the first stage of treatment in the month of remission induction, and this second half of this first in-patient phase was both easier and harder. Lauren was being given, relatively speaking, very little of the chemotherapy designed to kill the leukemia cells and so was in a recovering mode. This is the time when we watched a lot

---

14 By the end of the trip, because my temperature kept varying and this phenomenon had not been previously explained to us, I felt fine temperature-wise. I laughed and joked that we had all made the trip to Hamilton for nothing. I suggested that we go out for dinner. However, within a few minutes the fever was back. This was a strange time.

15 It was at this point that I became afraid that I had been misdiagnosed. I was shocked that I could get sick so quickly for no apparent reason once my diagnosis had been made. My dad encouraged me to ask the doctor about this and so I did. Subsequently, my doctor reassured me that I had the right diagnosis. However, she did not leave it at that. She wanted to truly convince me and so developed a plan. She got the slides of my biopsy and other slides to show me and compare. One afternoon I went down to the hematology lab and had a show of my own cancer cells. Here I was, face to face with my condition, the cancer cells so small, so weak looking, and ironically very beautiful. I could see what was wrong and what the problem was. This viewing, given by a sensitive doctor, changed my perspective on the control and elimination of my disease. Again, I knew it could and would be done.

of movies—many of them were for Lauren's film studies course, and Lauren worked on her magazine for children with cancer as a part of her creative writing course. After 10 more days in the hospital we went home for a few days before Lauren was to start the next stage of treatment—the prophylaxis and consolidation phase. These few days at home were an oasis. Lauren felt reasonably well and she had almost a normal amount of energy. I remember her working at her desk for a number of hours and going out to a debate and party on a weekend evening.

After 30 days, when the remission induction was complete and the remission was established with some near-normal blood counts, Lauren was to undergo 10 days of radiation to her head and four doses of intrathecal chemotherapy in her spine. This was to prevent the leukemia cells from lodging themselves in the cranium and proliferating there, as I understood it. Because there is a barrier between the brain and the rest of the bloodstream, the chemotherapy itself is not effective for the blood that circulates around the brain. In the early days of treatment for childhood leukemia, brain tumours would arise because the chemotherapeutically induced remission still left leukemia cells circulating in the brain.

We decided that rather than drive the hour or so from home each day in wintery weather we would stay at my brother's house, which was just about 15 minutes from the hospital where Lauren received her radiation and then just five minutes from where she received the intrathecal chemotherapy. My brother had lived away from Ontario for almost 20 years and so he had not been close to Lauren or Jess. This experience changed all that. We loved staying with Rich. He moved Lauren's mattress downstairs every morning so that she could watch videos and listen to music. He searched video stores for classic movies that he had enjoyed and wanted Lauren to see. He made wonderful bread, casseroles, salads, and (for me) coffee. He drove us every day to treatment.[16] By then I was a

---

16 Dad and Marian often came down to ride with us to radiation. This got to be a big occasion—all five of us driving to the clinic, stopping for my routine throwing up and then continuing on our way. These rides were very uncomfortable; radiation, funnily enough, was easier than the voyage there.

wreck, and so it was wonderful to have a driver and a caretaker. Lauren felt increasingly ill. As I recall, she was on ondonstetron all the time to minimize nausea. Still, we had fun and have memories of laughter, good talk, and wonderful home-made food. This is one of the times I am grateful for: through all the pain and suffering, new and deep human connections—uncle to niece, brother and sister—were cemented.[17]

We spent almost a month in the boot camp of the hospital. In some ways it seems a very short time. And, certainly it was a very short time to have had all those experiences. It also seems a very long time because so much happened and changed in our lives over that 30-day period. The rest of the treatment was essentially on an out-patient basis, although Lauren did have to be admitted once more while she decided whether to take the adriamyecin by bolus injection or infusion. (Bolus injection is a procedure in which the drug is pumped into the body over a short period of time—less than one hour while an out-patient in this case. Infusion would have taken 48 hours in the hospital.) That time, for two days, we shared a hospital room with a diabetic child with a cold. Lauren had the number of white cells thought to be enough to fight infection. Indeed, she did not get this cold, but it still troubled me to see such an incautious mix of patients. Lauren was also an in-patient later on at our local hospital, once for a period of two weeks when she had a fever above 38.5 and needed intravenous antibiotics. There were two other short stays to monitor and treat a fever. But this period I have just described at the teaching hospital took place over 30 days or so.

What do researchers say about the modern medical system and the modern hospital? What conclusions about bureaucracy and specialization do they draw? Are they inevitable in late modernity? Can

---

17 Uncle Richard, or Oily as I call him, was a godsend. He protected me and Mom. We talked for long times in the evenings. He gave his heart and energy to us for that three-week period and for this I will be eternally grateful. We always call my uncle the 'renaissance man', for he is an engineer, great chef, clarinet player, writer, and humorist. His house was a haven through a time in my life when I needed support walking, when I was too tired to talk or phone anyone, and when I physically felt like I was dying (although cognitively and emotionally I knew I was fine).

anything be done? The impact of health cuts on the suffering of sick people and those closest to them has not been the object of enough investigation. To combat the political-economic drive to 'claw back' moneys presently in the health-care system, substantial research documenting the real costs to both health-care providers and patients urgently needs to be done.

> **The Radiation Experience**
>
> I closed my eyes and
> darkness
> terror
> pain
> seized me
>
> I closed my eyes and
> panic
> looming
> suffocating
> overpowered me
>
> I closed my eyes and I
> couldn't move
> shouldn't move
> wouldn't move
>
> How do I describe radiation? For me, the first 10 seconds of treatment were probably the worst 10 seconds of my life. I thought that the room was pitch black, that if I opened my eyes I would see blinking lights and rays, and my eyes would be hurt. I thought that the smell that surrounded me was my skin burning. But, if I had opened my eyes I would have just seen the multimillion-dollar machine doing its job in a well-lit room. Also, the smell had nothing to do with me. It was the smell of ionizing oxygen, similar to the smell of lightning. My fears were unfounded.
>
> I had to wear a mask fitted to my head. It had taken three sessions to get it right, from the papier mâché stage to refitting it after I had cut

my hair. The mask was to keep my head in place and protect some parts of it while exposing others to the rays. This hard piece of plastic held me still so that I would be safe. I still have the mask. It is an extremely ugly, clear, inflexible piece of plastic. Red and blue lines mark its face. It has no resemblance to me. It is just a prop—but it still evokes anxiety in me.

The first time I was radiated, the nurse counted up from one to ten, then the radiation was over. This was supposed to relieve my fears, reassuring me that the time was almost finished. But as the number increased so did my level of tension. I could feel my breath quicken, my heart pounding, beating in my chest. After this experience, I knew that I couldn't go through it again without help.

That day, my family called everyone we knew to tell them how hard the radiation had been. We asked them to help me by praying and sending positive energy to me during my radiation session the next day.

At this same time, my uncle decided to do something concrete for me. My mom and I were being hosted magnificently by my uncle during my course of radiation. He would carry my mattress downstairs in the morning so I could lie around the house all day and then back up at night to sleep. He took care of my mom and me by driving us, making us wonderful meals, and by spending time with us. His life was put on hold for that month as well.

Early in my treatment, a friend had sent me the poem 'Invictus' by W.E. Henly. There is a line in it that states something to the effect of 'I am the master of my soul, I am the captain of my fate, my face may be bloodied, but I will continue on.' This poem inspired and comforted me. The feeling of not being in control of it all, yet needing to continue, needing to believe that I could choose to continue, was the key. I needed to have a sense of power somewhere. I was 'bloodied' and I was carrying on.

My uncle knew my feelings for this poem. He wrote a wonderful visualization for me about a female crane named Invicta. The crane was me. She was free and able to soar above it all in peace. She was alive and well.

The next morning, my second radiation treatment, the experience was radically different. I was calm going into the room. I was calm as I lay down on the metal bed. As they strapped my head in, I was able to

> breathe slowly and smile. Then, rather than the counting, my mom read the first paragraph of the visualization. I could see the crane soaring over the land. I tried to have my whole being in that flying.
>
> I didn't have the strength to go through these days alone, but with support I did. I drew on the power of all those who were thinking of me and the wonderful images that my uncle had so lovingly created.
>
> From *Imprint* (University of Waterloo), 31 Oct. 1997.

Our own experience in this system—of caring and occasionally careless medical personnel, of thoughtful and sometimes thoughtless interactions, of sensitivity and insensitivity, of waiting for desperate hours in emergency, of an infectious roommate and a mouse scurrying down a hospital hallway—is, I am sure, fairly typical. Except, perhaps, for one caveat: as a university professor, and a medical sociologist at that, I may have been advantaged by training and experience in terms of my interactions with medical personnel as the patient's parent and primary caregiver.

In any event, it was not an easy experience, and this is not an easy time to be caught up in the health-care system in Canada. I guess the excuse that could be offered is that this happened 'way back' in the mid-1990s, during a period of severe cut-backs in the health-care system. The significant political talk centred on such issues as deficit, debt, and their 'reduction', the Multilateral Agreement on Investment, and International Monetary Fund bailouts—with many strings attached—to debt-ridden countries. It was a time of the move to the right by North American governments. Since health care in Canada is largely public, the changes in government policy in Ontario had an immediate and dire impact on the day-to-day quality of health care in the province. But the same is true today, as even a casual glance at the daily newspapers will testify.

As George Torrance, one health policy analyst, has observed:

> The speed of change when it came in the late 1980's and especially in the 1990's was startling. The most dramatic manifestation is the closure of hospitals and beds in virtually all

provinces.... In Ontario, 20% of beds have been cut since 1986 and Metro Toronto has seen 30% closed or transformed. Between 1989 and 1994, Ontario closed 8,631 beds. On top of this, a report in the fall of 1995 recommended the closure of a dozen hospitals in Metro Toronto, reducing beds by 13%. The number of emergency rooms would be reduced from 21 to 14, the number of operating rooms from 184 to 154. (Torrance, 1998: 447)

As the bed numbers have declined, 'the number of patients treated actually increased—thanks to shorter stays and more day surgery and other outpatient services. The statistics tell the story. Over the past five years, day surgery procedures grew from about 750,000 to 925,000 a year. Acute care hospital beds in operation dropped by more than 5,000, and the average length of hospital stay fell from 8.7 to 7.2 days' (Armstrong and Armstrong, 1996:66). All this downsizing was accompanied, of course, by the lay-off of workers—nurses and nursing assistants—along with an increased reliance on part-time rather than full-time workers. Cost savings from using part-time workers result not only from the decrease in hours but also because it is not necessary to pay benefits to part-timers.

Table 3 portrays the extent of the cut-backs in hospitals in the period just before Lauren was diagnosed. Evidently, we experienced some of the effects of the cut-backs in sick and stressed nurses and doctors—and mice scampering around the floors.

Table 3
Staffed Beds in Hospitals, by Type of Care Unit, Canada and Provinces, 1986–7 and 1994–5.

	All units			Short-term care units			Long-term care units		
	1986–7	1994–5	% change	1986–7	1994–5	% change	1986–7	1994–5	% change
Canada*	172,425	120,774	-30.0	111,696	81,673	-26.9	60,729	39,101	-35.6
Newfoundland	3,401	2,753	-19.1	2,691	1,987	-26.2	710	766	-7.9
Prince Edward Island	755	513	-32.1	662	477	-27.9	93	36	-61.3
Nova Scotia	5,705	3,722	-34.8	5,242	3,324	-36.6	463	398	-14.0
New Brunswick	5,151	3,397	-34.1	3,949	2,494	-36.8	1,202	903	-24.9
Quebec	54,741	38,849	-29.0	27,089	25,121	-7.3	27,652	13,728	-50.4
Ontario	51,181	37,303	-27.1	37,334	24,354	-34.8	13,847	12,949	-6.5
Manitoba	6,369	5,527	-13.2	5,134	4,482	-12.7	1,235	1,045	-15.4
Saskatchewan	7,272	4,675	-35.7	6,448	4,097	-36.5	824	578	-29.9
Alberta	17,990	8,372	-53.5	11,755	7,598	-35.4	6,235	774	-87.6
British Columbia	19,466	15,527	-20.2	11,040	7,628	-30.9	8,426	7,899	-6.3

*Includes Northwest Territories and Yukon.
SOURCES: *Annual Return of Health Care Facilities—Hospitals, 1986/87*; *Preliminary Annual Report of Hospitals, 1994/95*. From Tully and Saint-Pierre, 1997.

Chapter 5

Mistakes Are Routine: Confusion, Contradiction, and the Unpredictable Cycle

Once the in-patient phase and the radiation and intrathecal treatments were completed, Lauren's treatment was to be as an out-patient. In our early innocence we thought that this would be lengthy and time-consuming, but we had not anticipated the interpersonal difficulties, the brutality of the health-care professionals at times, the continuing confusion and contradictions among different members of the health-care team, the competition between treatment centres, the reluctance to answer questions, the repeatedly changing faces and styles of residents, interns, and visiting doctors, the exhaustion from the weekly wait for treatment (to say nothing of that due to the medical treatment itself). In short, systemic, institutional, and interpersonal problems plagued the treatment cycle.

One of the chief continuing crises during Lauren's treatment was the contradictory, confusing, and sometimes clearly mistaken information we received. The first example I have already described—the resident who said that Lauren would lose 10 IQ points, as if it were inevitable, after radiation to her head. A second 'mistake' was one made very early in the treatment by Lauren's 'own' out-patient nurse. She said that Lauren had been selected at random for a bolus infusion of adriamyecin (which we came to call 'adria') rather than a 48-hour infusion of the drug. She presented this as a good thing. It meant that she wouldn't have to be hospitalized for 48 hours every three weeks. Instead, she would be injected with adriamyecin over a period of one-half hour every three weeks. We rejoiced—until that date of the first appointment.

During the course of the discussions about this next stage of treatment and the scheduling of her weekly treatments Dr M, one of the pediatric oncologists in this hospital, raised the topic of the 'adria' injection. He said that Lauren had been randomized into the

48-hour continuous infusion option and that she would be admitted to the hospital immediately after the morning clinic. And so I had to say, 'Oh no, she is randomized into the bolus. K told us and I have it underlined by K in one of the sheets of paper that we received that explained the treatment protocol'. But the doctor reiterated, 'I have it here, direct from the principal investigator of the study. Lauren is on 48-hour infusion'. He left the room, double-checked, and came back to us to repeat once again his opinion.

I instantly knew that he had all the power and that we needed to forget what we had been told, and told with enthusiasm, by Lauren's nurse earlier. I asked, 'If Lauren is randomized into the 48-hour protocol infusion, what might the benefits to her be?' It was clear that 48 hours in hospital every three weeks was definitely going to be costly to her 'quality of life' over the next period of approximately 10 months while undergoing this first and most aggressive stage of out-patient treatment. He said that he didn't know what its advantage might be for her, a fully grown 17-year-old, because the research was on children of an average age of four years who had been treated for leukemia 20 years previously. However, researchers and clinicians were finding that these kids, now in their middle twenties, often seemed to have irregular heart rhythms. They hadn't found heart disease, but there was a tendency to abnormal heart rhythms.

I said that I knew that 'adria' had been used in the treatment of adults with cancer for many years, and asked if research on adults had been found to be related to heart problems of any sort. The doctor responded, I thought, angrily and sarcastically: 'No—they all die!' Questions and tough, educated discussion apparently were unacceptable and off limits. And so I said to myself I wasn't going to get any further with this conversation and concluded immediately that I needed to appear to acquiesce to his opinion.

The clinic had two pharmacists who were part of the 'team' at the time. After the meeting with the pediatric oncologist I asked one of the pharmacists to do some research (it seemed a practical and good use of her skills to me) on adriamyecin by injection infusion as compared to bolus in adults so that Lauren could decide whether or not it would be worth her while to remain in hospital for this particular treatment every three weeks. In the meantime, for the first cycle we stayed in hospital so that Lauren could have the 48-hour infusion, keep her options open, and remain in the protocol to which she was apparently randomized.[1]

Within two weeks the pharmacist had good news for us, news about which she was very excited. As she understood it from the literature, 'adria', when injected, caused a sudden increase in the speed of the pumping of the heart. The 48-hour infusion, because it would spread out the impact of the drug, would minimize this dramatic impact. But she knew that hospitalization was also an issue for Lauren and she had found a further exciting piece of news.

There was a study, out of Chicago as I recall, in which the drug was pumped over 48 hours by a portable pump that was attached to the body through a 'port' (or port-a-cath). This is an implanted catheter that provides a very effective means for allowing entry into the large veins for chemotherapy, intravenous fluids, antibiotics, blood and platelet transfusions, blood taking, and IV nutrition. With the exception of IV nutrition, all of these are recurrent treatments for a child with cancer. A port-a-cath would allow Lauren complete mobility. It had never been used with children as far as she knew. She thought that she could find a pump in the hospital and convince the team to let Lauren try it, if Lauren wanted to do so. We talked briefly and Lauren said yes—the risks were minimal and the benefits were maximal. So Lauren became a maverick, receiving her 'adria' by portable pump over 48 hours every three weeks (this cycle turned out to be only theoretical, as you will learn soon). She was thus able to go to school, maintain some of her social life, and stay out of the hospital. She wore the pump around

---

1 I found out about this negative (to my lifestyle) change of plans at a very inopportune time. Dr M announced that I was in remission—a cause for tremendous celebration. Then, within almost the same breath, he told me that I had a room in the ward and could start the next part of treatment immediately. What a let-down! I was ready to go home (I had been planning to) and celebrate with family and friends, and now I was being told that I had to stay for two days in the hospital, not my favourite vacation spot. We quickly decided to stay, to buy more time, but negotiated to be able to leave for a lunch out that I had been looking forward to. Unfortunately, the premeds I was given before departure made me drowsy and spacey, so the lunch was not very memorable. In fact, I almost felt like passing out.

her waist and the tube attachment was under her clothes and inserted into her 'port'. It looked like a money belt for a kid on her way to summer in Europe.[2]

When Lauren was diagnosed the doctor had said that her treatment would be two years in length. The two-year plan of treatment was divided into stages. The first stage was the remission induction, during which the aim was to kill as many leukemia cells as possible and establish a remission of the disease for Lauren. A number of different drugs were used in this stage: dexamethasone, vincristine, intrathecal ARA-C or cytarbine, adriamyecin, methotrexate, and citrovorum. This stage lasted the first month. The second stage was called the CNS (central nervous system) prophylaxis and intensification stage. Over a period of 51 weeks Lauren was to be on a three-week cycle that included initially 10 days of cranial radiation, four days of intrathecal methotrexate and ARA-C (these were the CNS prophylaxis treatments designed to prevent the spread of the leukemia cells to the brain). Every three weeks over the next 51 weeks, Lauren was to receive vincristine, 6-mercaptopurine, L'asparaginese, adriamyecin, and dexamethasone. All of these drugs were to be given every third week with the exception of L'asparaginese. This was administered weekly, via a needle in Lauren's upper leg. The final stage was called maintenance. From week 53 to the end, Lauren was to receive, again on tri-weekly and weekly cycles, vincristine, dexamethasone, methotrexate, and 6-mercaptopurine. We quickly learned that the three-week cycle was a myth, a mirage. The weekly injection of L-asparaginese occurred rain or shine, with one hour of blood-pressure reading afterwards. It did not require adequate blood counts. However, 'week one', which was the first week of the tri-weekly schedule for the rest of the drugs, almost never occurred on schedule, at least not for Lauren.

As well as chemotherapy every week, Lauren had to have regular weekly blood counts. Her blood-count level determined

---

2 This 'money belt' let me be free, period. I always loved to explain to others what was happening to me, if they asked. Whenever I wore the pump to school someone would want to see it. I was glad to do this, for I felt that making my treatment as normal to others as possible would allow them to see me as the 'same old Lauren' more easily and not be fearful of contact.

whether or not she would receive treatment as well as the quantity of the various drugs. Both the calculations and the cut-off points were somewhat idiosyncratic in regard to when treatment would be delayed—they varied from treatment centre to treatment centre and from research study to research study. In fact, the calculations and cut-off points changed at least once during the treatment. There were three significant readings—hemoglobin, white blood count (WBC), and platelets—but there were a number of components. The WBC seemed to be most affected by the chemotherapy, which was designed, if that word can be used for something similar to the design of the fallout of a nuclear bomb, to depress the functioning of the bone marrow and to kill any leukemic cells in the bloodstream.

In any case, as soon as Lauren's first cycle rolled around we realized we had 'failed'. Her 'counts' were not high enough. Her white blood count was less than required. She was neutropenic and lacked the necessary ingredients to fight infection. The unspoken message in all this was (to us) that Lauren's body was failing the protocol. I knew and she knew and all of those who cared most deeply knew—failure to have a high white blood count meant a failure to follow the protocol and also meant to us an unmentionable possibility, failure to survive.[3] No one ever said exactly what it was, but I guessed there was a cut-off point after which Lauren would no longer be a part of the 'successful' protocol that she had agreed to be part of.

Whose mistake was this? Should they have told us that the cycle of chemotherapy was idealized? Should they have told us that no one—or a few, about half, most but not all, or whatever the statistics are—is able to receive chemotherapy on schedule ... or was it our mistake? I discovered at the end of her treatment, through aggressively pursuing the question of whether or not Lauren's treatment was finished, that only 1 to 2 per cent of all those to have been treated according to this protocol were able to receive all the required drugs on schedule. This figure was based on all the 700-

---

3   For me, the protocol was not such an important goal. I was going to survive, no matter what drugs I took or did not take. This was always a given for me throughout treatment.

plus children in Canadian and US sites who had been enrolled in this particular protocol since 1985. It would have been very helpful to have known this early in Lauren's treatment. It would have saved us from considerable anxiety. Whenever she was unable to receive chemotherapy I felt a failure as a mother, protector, and caretaker, and I expect she felt this even more strongly.[4]

I was totally unprepared for the situation in which her counts weren't high enough. We had no forewarning that this was a possibility. When this continued not just for one week but for two and then three, we were not only ill-prepared but concerned, worried, anxious, fearful, and confused.[5] What did this mean? Her prognosis was based on regular chemotherapy and now she wasn't getting it. One didn't have to spend much time thinking through the situation to hypothesize that the prognosis must be changing. And likely not for the best. For every week that Lauren missed her chemotherapy was she losing 1 per cent, 10 per cent, 20 per cent, or what probability of survival? This was a very anxious time. Especially so because in the middle of this, three young people within our small world of illness and survival—a daughter of a sports star, the son of a fellow out West who had protested in front of the government offices in the hopes that his son could be treated with new and experimental treatment available only in the US, and the little girl in the hospital room beside Lauren—died.

What else could we do? I talked with friends of a friend whose son had received treatment at the same centre a few years before. These parents, both of whom were physicians, had a number of

---

4   I think in the beginning I felt like I had failed somehow. But quite quickly this was replaced with another feeling—that of separation from my body. It was not me who was sick, but my body; I was not the low blood counts—my bone marrow was producing them. I took care of myself as best as I could, and inherently I knew my body was doing the same for itself. Like the weeds that grow out of cement, my body is made to survive and thus would survive. I have had an amazing awakening to awe for my body, for all of our bodies and the earth around us, through this experience. I often marvel at how strong I am now and that my body could heal. There is much wonder in our world.

5   I don't remember fear. I had faith in my body to heal itself with some help. At the beginning (the first five, six months or so) I was too sick to think about getting better or getting worse. After this point my strength and weight (I had lost 30 pounds) started to increase and I felt healthy. I was more frustrated by the lack of treatment than scared.

things to say, one of which was to suggest that I ask the doctors if they had thought that G-CSF (granulocyte colony-stimulating factor) might have a role in the treatment of leukemia. They said it was new but that the research literature on it seemed to indicate that it was very promising for raising white blood counts. It provided a sort of immune system therapy. It reduced neutropenia and thus had been found to keep people out of the hospital with the fevers and infections that often accompanied neutropenia. The fact that it kept people out of the hospital made it a fairly successful drug. It was, however, very expensive. Patent protection enabled the manufacturer to keep the cost up to about $150 per day.[6]

The next week when we went to the hospital we asked the doctor about the role of G-CSF. He said they didn't use it with leukemia. And I said that I would afford it. At the end of this clinic visit we asked the pharmacist about G-CSF and leukemia. We wondered what the problems were, why wasn't it used. He replied that they only used it in extreme cases and that we should ask Lauren's doctor and not him. We had thought that the pharmacist knew more about specific pharmaceuticals, their effects and side-effects, and had access to the most up-to-date reliable research literature. We had thought that was why they had hired this expert with a Ph.D. in pharmacology. However, without any explanation as to the rationale for the change, the next week Lauren's doctor said that he had ordered G-CSF for Lauren. In the meantime, I had a 20-page Internet search in my briefcase, which included some research studies describing G-CSF and its use with leukemia. I was glad to be able to keep it in my briefcase, but at the same time the process of successfully advocating for a drug that had at first been rejected by the experts—the pediatric oncologist and pharmacist—left me feeling more and more insecure about the treatment protocol that Lauren was part of, about the knowledge of the medical team, and ultimately, which was surely the only thing of final importance to me, about Lauren's treatment and her well-being.

Lauren started on neupogen (the G-CSF). Her counts were

---

6 This treatment, like ondonsetron, was only available to me because both my parents had very high medical coverage. I was lucky.

expected to go down 7–10 or 14 days after the various drugs that she was on. Thus, it was suggested that she go on G-CSF on the 15th to 21st day of each month. This, it was hoped, would bring her counts (WBC) up high enough to get the chemotherapy that would put her counts back down again 10–14 days later. This first cycle of G-CSF didn't raise her counts high enough and so this medication was continued until the next week, when she was able to submit to the whole arsenal again.[7] On the next cycle the WBC (on which the G-CSF worked and which had been the problem in previous stages of her cycle) was okay but the platelets were not. So again she had to wait. I later discovered that there had been an ongoing experimental use of neupogen (G-CSF) at another teaching hospital with a pediatric oncology unit. Here it had been determined that neupogen did raise the white blood cell count, but because both platelets and WBC originated in the same stem cell, whenever the white blood cell count increased the platelet count was likely to decrease.

The reverse Russian roulette continued. More times than not Lauren was not able to get her drugs on the prescribed day of the prescribed week, and so it and our anxiety continued from week to week and cycle to cycle. Our having been prepared to expect a three-week cycle, this on-again, off-again process played havoc with my emotions. Every time it didn't happen 'as it was supposed to', I had to get up the courage to problem-solve, look at the Internet, call around the country to treatment centres, call on friends for advice, and confront the doctors with questions and demands. I can't help but think that it would have been helpful to have known initially that the cycle was a mirage, an ideal chimera, and that it was normal to miss some cycles of treatment.[8]

---

7   G-CSF was a bitter drug to take. Although I always wanted as much chemotherapy as I could get, part of me questions the fact that we overruled my body's response. It was clearly saying 'too much', yet we said 'take more!' Who was right? There is no answer to this question, except the fact that, regardless, I am here today.

8   It seems to me that this mirage was truly pointless. If they wanted a placebo effect (a belief that I would get chemotherapy every three weeks), it didn't work. In fact, the negative effect of worry and fear on the part of my parents, and on my part, too, I'm sure worsened my day-to-day health. If one thing should be told to parents and patients at

All of these inconsistencies about the cycle seem to me to be even more problematic and even ironic because of an interaction between Dr M and Lauren in December, to which I was a helpless bystander. Earlier in November, just after Lauren's 12 October diagnosis, her dad had discussed scheduling Lauren's chemotherapy so that she could feel as well as possible during the upcoming Christmas holiday. Richard asked, with all of our agreement, that her chemotherapy be moved back a day per cycle until Christmas to enable her to feel okay at this time and then to miss school on Fridays for clinic on a regular basis rather than some other school day, come the new term in January. Dr M and Lauren's dad had worked out that change quite amicably.[9] It didn't seem to be a problem. But we rethought it and decided that the first plan was actually the best for Lauren and, on our own, we informed the nurses that we would be coming in for the originally scheduled day. No one objected or said it was a problem.

Later, when we met with the doctor again he noticed that the change had been made and shouted angrily at Lauren that she was not to change the schedule on her own and that such changes could kill her, that her specific and timely treatment was a matter of life and death. Lauren was humiliated and devastated.[10] I was furious. However, because we were so afraid of this aggressive man—who had previously said that adults with cancer couldn't be looked to for information about the impact of adriamyecin on the heart because they all died—and in such a vulnerable position, we apologized and took responsibility for the mistake.

---

    the commencement of chemo it is that each body responds differently to everything—the drugs, the possible side-effects, the decor in the treatment waiting room.

9 This is important to note. If I wanted something arranged with Dr M, I would always ask my dad to do the arranging. Dr M, from the beginning, epitomized to me the patronizing, patriarchal, archetypical doctor. In responding to me or my female relatives, my mom primarily, he was hard-pressed to find the easy jocularity that he reserved for the males. This experience ran contrary to what I had been expecting. Early in my treatment a young man had come to talk to me. He had said that Dr M was his favourite doctor. This was not the case for this educated, confident young woman.

10 In fact, I broke down in tears. Dr M did nothing. He just continued his tirade and then went on to other issues—all because my dad had used 10 minutes of his time discussing a slight diversion from the already random protocol.

In actuality, the doctor was wrong in a number of ways, I think. It was Lauren's dad, Richard, with whom he had made the contract to change the schedule—not Lauren. It was Richard to whom he should have spoken. Lauren was not a free agent in any of this. She was very sick at the time and she was not able to drive to appointments by herself. The other issue is that this sort of aggressively barbarian behaviour frightened us, in itself, and heightened any fear we had about Lauren's treatment protocol and the extent to which this doctor, in particular, cared about her at all.

I doubt that anyone would think that such cruelty is an acceptable interpersonal style in any interaction. In the interaction between a very sick and vulnerable teenage girl and her doctor it is especially outlandish. One doesn't expect health-care providers to be abusive or brutish in their interactions with ill people. There is certainly no evidence that this type of bedside manner is associated with better health outcomes.

Considerable research suggests that positive and supportive relationships are fundamental to good health. (See, for example, the study done by Spiegal [1991], which demonstrates the survival benefits of group support for women diagnosed with metastatic breast cancer.) This behaviour cannot possibly be seen as promoting health. Why did we experience such destructive hostility from this doctor? Was it just him, his personality? Had we aggravated him sufficiently in our several conflictual interactions to merit such a response? Was he suffering from stress as the result of the cut-backs that had occurred at the clinic in the previous few years? How can we understand such behaviour? How can we explain the problems that the doctors were faced with that led them to be less than they could have and perhaps would have liked to be? Some research literature suggests that the lot of the doctors in modern society is not a happy one. While their physical health tends to surpass the physical health of the general population, their mental health falls below (Ramirez et al., 1995). The suicide rates among doctors are relatively high. Some researchers have found that doctors, along with other health-care providers, tend to suffer burnout related to the stressfulness of their work (Freudenberger, 1974). Among doctors, moreover, there is some evidence that those who work primarily with people with cancer are particularly susceptible to work-related stresses and dissatisfaction (Delvaux et al., 1988). A series of studies have found psychiatric disorder in almost one-third of this population. Ramirez et al. (1995) found the rate of psychiatric disorder, as determined by scores on the well-validated General Health Questionnaire, to be 28 per cent. Among the most significant sources of stress for the doctors in the study included: (1) feeling overworked and the effect of this on home life, (2) organizational conflicts and responsibilities, (3) dealing with a patient's suffering, and (4) being involved with treatment toxicity and errors.

Lauren's diagnosis in 1995 in Ontario occurred at a time of Draconian cutbacks in the health-care system in general, with the closing down of hospitals, wards, beds, and special services (as described in the previous chapter). In the particular unit in which Lauren was diagnosed and treated the number of oncologists declined by 33 per cent within the first month after diagnosis and never (over her treatment period) increased again.

Another one of the ways that researchers have attempted to understand the working life of doctors and nurses is through the concept of burnout. This concept positions the health-care provider as an occupant of a particular job or a particular organization suffering from some of the exigencies of the working life.

Burnout has been defined as follows: 'to fail, wear out, or become exhausted by making excessive demands on energy, strength, or resources' (Freudenberger, 1974: 159). It is said that burnout may be a problem for people in particularly demanding occupations. Often, those who are the most dedicated and committed are the ones who experience burnout.[11] Signs of the problem include various and frequently intractable physical symptoms, such as a lingering cold, recurrent headaches, or sleeplessness. Often, there are behavioural accompaniments, including 'quickness

---

11 I am not a psychologist, but this would seem to fit some of Dr M's behaviours. I knew that he was very skilled technically (successful bone marrow aspiration and spinal taps prove this). Also, he is humorous and well liked by some patients. He is on many boards dealing with pediatric oncology. However, the feeling of being seen as too assertive (I believe, in particular, because Mom and I are both female) was palpable.

to anger' and 'instantaneous irritation and frustration' (ibid., 160). Thinking may become 'rigid, stubborn and inflexible'. According to Maslach and Jackson (1986), who developed a scale for its measurement, burnout is typified by emotional exhaustion, depersonalization, and a diminished sense of accomplishment. Further, they argue, it is particularly endemic among health professionals and other occupational groups who work with people.

Such responses may be particularly evident among physicians, and especially among oncologists (Whippen and Canellos, 1991). Burnout is notably associated with health-care work: 'the end result of stress in the professional life of a physician or care giver [is] apathy, suspicion, self-protection, disillusion, and depression' (ibid., 1916). Whippen and Canellos studied a random sample of 1,000 physicians who subscribed to the *Journal of Clinical Oncology*. The overall response rate, without any reminders or other follow-up, was a very respectable 60 per cent. Of the 598 respondents, 56 per cent reported some degree of burnout related to their work. More recent graduates had a higher likelihood of burnout than earlier graduates: 67 per cent of those who had graduated since 1980, as compared to 47 per cent and 48 per cent of those who had graduated prior to 1970 and between 1970 and 1979. Interestingly, then, oncologists were not more likely to experience burnout as the result of longer years on the job. Working outside of a clinic or university structure seemed to lead to a greater probability of burnout. One of the major reasons for the feeling of burnout was insufficient vacation or personal time (57 per cent). Other factors were continuous exposure to terminal illness (53 per cent) and frustration with therapeutic outcomes. The researchers concluded as follows: 'burnout can be seen not as a condemnation of the professional activity per se but rather a reflection of the total quantity of the emotional stresses of practice, which dominate the majority of professional time in the practice of oncology' (ibid., 1920).

All interpersonal work involves some management of emotional labour (Hochschild, 1979, 1983). Medical work is no exception. In fact, it could be argued that medical work, particularly the practice of oncology, demands a great deal of emotional work because of the solemn nature of the typical diagnosis and prognosis. Doctors, more than most others, interact with people in the rawest of situations. They must see and work with the naked body, and must deal with terror, fear, disappointment, and anger in the face of a serious diagnosis, and even must cope at times with rage from the patient and the patient's family when the doctor is unable to effect a cure. In spite of the extremely traumatic situations within which doctors must work, they are expected to control their expression of emotions and to treat all patients in exactly the same way (Parsons, 1951, 1954). Regardless of their feelings, they are expected to manifest a 'cloak of competence' (Haas and Shaffir, 1977), and in the face of unsettling feelings doctors must learn to manage their emotions. Yet they are not taught emotion management in medical school or on the job.

Smith and Kleinman (1989) interviewed and observed medical students over a period of two years as they encountered the human body through the dissection of cadavers and the execution of pelvic examinations, two of the most 'intimate' of the approaches that students and then physicians make to the human body. The purpose of these observations and subsequent interviews was to describe how physicians in training learned to handle the emotions that arose in these situations. They found that there are different strategies and that they reflect the culture of modern Western medicine.

The fundamental strategy used is analytic transformation. This essentially involved transforming the contact from one with a human being to one with a body, a body part, or a problem. This serves to provide distance from the patient. It also enables the students to focus on redefining the contact as good because it reflects 'real medicine'. After years of anticipation, they could say to themselves that they were actually entering the profession because they were focused on malfunctioning bodies and how to fix them. They were able to do this inasmuch as they maintained power over the patient so that the patient did not become a person, an equal. At the same time, doctors-in-training are taught to be somewhat empathetic with patients, though not too much so. 'Students are taught that excessive concern for patients can cloud their clinical judgment, but moderate concern allows them to manage their own feelings and to pay close attention to the patient' (Smith and Kleinman,

1989: 67). Humour is another emotion management tactic used in these circumstances. By redefining an aspect of the situation or problem as humorous, the medical students were able to distance themselves and handle the challenges.

Frederick Hafferty is another researcher who has looked at the emotional labour involved in doctoring. His focus was on the role of humour, particularly what he calls cadaver stories, defined 'as narratives describing "jokes" played by medical student protagonists on unsuspecting and emotionally vulnerable victims' (Hafferty, 1988: 344). Humour, in this context, is a way of coping with the onslaught of emotion that might otherwise result from the life-and-death intensity of (some) medical work. His observation is that cadaver stories are an essential part of the oral culture of medical training.

Another technique for emotional coping is the avoidance of contact. The use of various drapes and covers assists in this process. Through their study and practice, students gradually come to view the human body as an interesting object, separate from the person. The body becomes an intellectual construct that is (relatively) stripped of cultural metaphors and meaning. Hafferty's study corresponds in some ways to the literature and research on burnout, in that it shows how burnout, in particular, depersonalization, is an adaptive strategy that may be used by doctors to manage their emotions. Becoming desensitized is a crucial part of becoming a doctor. It is not appropriate for a doctor to respond sexually when doing a pelvic examination; it is not appropriate for a doctor to respond with sobbing when announcing bad news. Doctors must eventually learn to protect themselves and to do the emotion work involved in the management of feelings that has been described.

However, and for whatever series of reasons, some of Lauren's doctors were not always able to manage their emotions and they spilled over onto Lauren and us, her family members. This was often hurtful. Another explanation for this brutal response may be that I violated the well-entrenched norm in the relations between medical doctors and patients (and family members of patients)—the norm of asymmetry. Doctors are presumed to be in control and have been shown to work to maintain control over the talk that occurs with patients. The position of the patient has been described as one of 'interactional submission'. There is asymmetry of topic, 'in the sense that it is the patient's condition that is under review rather than the doctor's' (Pilnick, 1998: 31).

I have described how I had to ask several health-care professionals to leave our hospital room. I have also described confusion, contradiction, tactlessness, and medical errors in the care that Lauren received from health-care professionals. What is the role of a parent in these situations? How can parents intervene in ways that protect their children? Lozowski et al. (1993: 64) reported on a study of parental intervention in medical care. They assert that childhood cancer is very stressful in itself, but they also make the point that 'the medical staff can help exacerbate or mediate such stress and have a major impact on the parents' views about the quality of care they and their children receive.' I would have to agree that the medical staff, at times, exacerbated the stress of the disease. It is inevitable, to some extent, that conflicts would occur between and among parents, ill children, and some of the variety of health-care providers. After all, the relationship is non-voluntary. Children do not choose to become ill. Health-care providers do not have the luxury of choosing to work with the patients they like while avoiding others. Both parties are involuntarily associated with one another. Moreover, these relationships, in the case of a chronic illness or a disease such as childhood cancer, may last over a lengthy period of time. In addition, the relationships are to some extent and in some ways intimate relationships. Certainly in a physical sense, the health-care providers have intimate access to the vulnerable body and emotions of the sick.

All of us make errors. I have made many spelling and grammatical errors, even in the shortest and simplest of words and sentences, as I have been writing this book. I have also made more serious errors in more important parts of my life. Health-care providers also make errors—technical, interpersonal, moral, and other errors (Millman, 1977). When parents are in the hospital alongside their children they are likely to observe a few or more than a few errors. However, 'responding to or acting to prevent apparent errors challenges these norms of compliance with expert authority and goes beyond the suggestions of most professionals regarding parental activism and involvement' (Lozowski et al., 1993: 66).

Some researchers who have studied and written about parental involvement outside of the strictly parental tasks such as feeding, dressing, preparing, and calming the child for treatment tend to disparage parental involvement by characterizing it as indicative of a 'struggle for control' (Kirkpatrick, Hoffman, and Futterman, 1974). Mattson (1979: 259) went further and suggested that parents who are under stress may act out their fears and anger by attacking staff and challenging them in an irrational manner: 'they may displace and project helpless and angry feelings about their child's condition onto various medical professionals, and blame them for delays and mistakes in treating the child.'

This may occur at times, but there are also many important instances of beneficial parental involvement. Barbarin and Chesler (1986: 234) noted that '[e]merging trends in the treatment of childhood cancer, such as the skyrocketing financial burden on parents, increased life expectancy and reliance on outpatient treatment, are likely to increase the need for parents to monitor medical and psychosocial services and to provide additional care over an extended time period.' In the research of Lozowski et al. (1993: 73) on parents of children with cancer the following types of parental intervention were reported:

> Patient as expert—the parent corrected the staff regarding details about the patient's care that the staff did not know[12]—interpersonal negotiator—parent intervened because of staff's attitude or style—monitor IV procedures—parent intervened regarding problems specifically related to IV procedures—procedure historian—parent called staff's attention to incorrect or excessive procedures—rescuer—parent intervened to keep staff from giving patient the wrong treatment or an excessive amount of a drug.

---

12 Many times I was asked what drugs I needed. We have arranged all my out-patient visits. I self-monitored my pill-taking (even self-injecting neupogen) as soon as I was able. Much of the associated work around illness takes place away from the clinic. Without the consent and active participation of the patient (and in the case of children, parents) treatment would not work.

Their data show 'that parental intervention in treatment, at least in this study population, was fairly common' and that parents' decisions to intervene were not made easily. Instead, many parents carefully considered the ramifications of intervening. Many reported that they were intimidated by the staff and therefore reluctant to assert themselves. They were concerned about 'being viewed as overassertive or aggressive, behaving in ways that might be construed as negative or overly critical, or being perceived as overprotective of their child.... They often reported being afraid that if they made a fuss, their child might suffer and receive less attention, less empathic care, and the like' (ibid., 79, 80, 81).[13] However, they found that parents with higher income and education levels were more likely to intervene. In addition, with a status closer to that of the medical professionals who were caring for their child, these parents may have felt freer to challenge their 'status peers'.

Such inferences are confirmed by Cockerham (1988), who reported that usually the poor tended to be relatively passive recipients of professional health services and were more likely to invest responsibility for their own health in the health-care system than in themselves. Barbarin and Chesler (1986) found that less educated parents were 'less likely to question the authority or judgment of doctors'. At the same time, married people and those involved in support groups were more likely to intervene than single and divorced parents.

Parents who intervened generally tended to express less satisfaction with the emotional support provided by staff. Barbarin and Chesler, who conducted an interview study with 74 parents from 45 families with children living with cancer, offer a viewpoint that may aid in understanding our troubled experiences with the medical care team at the teaching hospital. They found that doctors and other medical staff had much poorer relationships with parents

---

13 I remember having this feeling. The sentiment of 'let's not rock the boat' would ring through my head over my mom's interventions at times. Sometimes I think she reacted better than I would have, and at other times I think we could have let things go. But who is to say? Why should asking polite questions make anyone respond so negatively, as we sometimes found? Obviously, there was something wrong with the respondent or the situation she or he was in.

who were assertive, asked questions, and were 'more information-seeking, more problem-solving', and less likely to deny. Parents with passive and acquiescent coping strategies were likely to have better relationships with the medical staff. In addition, they found that the more assertive parents tended to be the more educated parents. They speculate, 'Because parents with higher levels of education are closer to the professional status of the medical staff they may be less willing to be compliant and to "sit still" in the face of questionable staff behaviors and attitudes. Perhaps, too, they are more likely to see clearly and discuss openly the uncertain grounds on which all treatment for cancer rests' (Barbarin and Chesler, 1986: 233).

It is impossible for me to know how my attitudes and behaviour, as a relatively educated, single, middle-aged person, compared to those of other, younger, perhaps less educated fathers and mothers. I do not know what I might have done or said that would have proven to be particularly threatening. I am obviously just a case of one and cannot generalize from my experience. Nevertheless, I would like to note that my difficult relationships were both infrequent in the big city hospital (although very troubling)[14] and did not continue over into the local community hospital, where I was always able to ask questions and be involved in decisions without seeming to threaten what turned out to be an excellent ongoing relationship with the pediatricians and nurses.

---

14 My experience while under primary care was not all bad. Truly, there were many people who helped: Dr Q, clinic nurses, the teacher, the first resident, many, many of my day/night nurses, the radiation nurse. However, a few instances, like the radiation resident, my 'dressing down' by Dr M, and the sick nurses cloud my perception of my time there. What went wrong should not have happened. I am thankful to those who did help and were supportive.

Chapter 6

Clinic Visits: Here or There?

The out-patient phase had been described to us as a weekly visit to the clinic at the teaching hospital, which was about an hour away, where Lauren would receive her treatment, be examined by the doctor, and have time to visit with 'her' nurse. This was to take place over approximately two years.

The hour drive to the clinic for the weekly treatments began during the winter when the roads were often bad and the drive was treacherous. The clinic wait was always all morning. Even without treatment Lauren was never finished before 11 a.m., and usually it was after 1 p.m. before we could leave.[1] We seemed to always be the last to leave even though we were often the first to arrive. During the time that Lauren was still in the hospital her nurse had recommended that Lauren avoid the long wait at the clinic by aiming to be there by 10 a.m. rather than at 8:30 a.m. when the 'finger poke' nurse was ready to take blood. A few times we tried to use Lauren's nurse's advice to arrive late, for about 10. It didn't ever help the sequencing of the treatment. In fact, Lauren was scolded several times by one of the other four nurses on duty for coming late. This seemed particularly unnecessary, as Lauren wasn't a free agent in her attendance at the clinic—she was too sick to drive herself and, also, I wanted to be with her. Her father usually had to work, but Marian almost always drove down so that I could be free if Lauren needed anything on the trip.

---

1   I accept all of these as possible reasons for our seeking another out-patient clinic. Also, the fact that I did not go to the teaching hospital clinic often later meant that the staff and I did not get to know each other very well. However, the feeling of neglect and indifference came long before we decided to change hospitals. There is no conflict about the chicken and the egg. If we had been happy with the atmosphere, interpersonal care, and structure of the first hospital, we would have stayed.

The clinic wait was not fun! Early on Lauren felt very sick and had to get up early to be in the car to arrive at the hospital, go by wheelchair to the clinic, and then lie on a couch in the waiting room or, eventually, on a bed in the clinic, feeling terrible while little kids played, watched TV, and were visited by the child-life team or the various volunteers. Because Lauren had agreed to be part of a research study on the impact of physical activity on her health during and after treatment, the physiotherapist often visited.[2]

But given the long wait, the indifference and even nasty conflicts involved in a few of the interactions with the clinic nurses and doctors, the frequent absence of 'her' nurse, the plethora of small children, many with colds, and the long drive over winter roads, when we found there was a local out-patient pediatric oncology clinic about five minutes from our house we were thrilled. Our home-care nurse, having known about the local clinic, had given us information and checked to see that they were able to do Lauren's required treatments. We decided to visit the clinic, to find out if it would be any better, or at least as good, and to see whether or not Lauren could get her treatments there.

The nurses at the local clinic seemed very warm and knowledgeable. One had a great deal of experience, over 10 years at a major teaching hospital in pediatric oncology, and the other had several years of experience. They said that they would gladly take Lauren into their care on an out-patient basis. The pediatrician who was in charge of the clinic was well respected by the nurses and, although not a hemotologist or oncologist, had worked with pediatric oncology protocols over a number of years.

Lauren decided that it was appealing to move to the local hospital. The next obstacle to surmount was to get approval for this change from the primary-care clinic. This was a major blockade. No one in the teaching hospital had ever mentioned community-based pediatric oncology outpatient treatment centres to us. However,

---

2   The physiotherapist was one of the most responsive people at the clinic. She would always check in on me and see how I was progressing. She was proud of my regaining strength. She also seemed to have a pretty realistic view of my progress and this was helpful. I didn't feel like I was ever failing in our interviews.

the people in our local hospital clinic worked with staff from two other major teaching hospitals with pediatric oncology centres. They were highly experienced in the administration of the drugs and in troubleshooting any unusual problems during treatment for childhood cancers. Still, we were fearful about asking. When we first mentioned the possibility we were told it was not done. I talked to one nurse on my own and she suggested that it might be in Lauren's best interest to have her care consolidated at the teaching hospital because they had all the specialists available—child-life workers, physiotherapists, chaplains, social workers, nurses, doctors, interns, residents, visiting doctors, and volunteers. Still another nurse implied that the move was for my convenience, not Lauren's, because Lauren would need the psychosocial support they were able to offer. But we persevered.[3]

Despite the resistance of the teaching hospital pediatric oncology team, by mid-January they had reluctantly agreed and Lauren was receiving her treatment locally for two of three weeks. We felt that Lauren was in good hands medically. It turned out that the psychosocial experience at the local clinic was immeasurably better. Lauren developed very positive, supportive relationships with the nurses and with the doctors, particularly the chief pediatrician. As did I.

That is not to say that the next two years were easy, but at this particular clinic the suffering was due to the necessary medical treatments and not to churlishness and confusion. Lauren and I

---

3   And to paraphrase Robert Frost, 'this is what made all the difference.' Rather than spending every full Friday driving to the out-of-town hospital, missing the day of school (first high school, then university), and becoming exhausted (always the result of an out-of-town clinic visit), we would be spending five minutes driving and at the most an hour and a half at the local clinic. Thus I could go to school in the morning and clinic in the afternoon. The assertion that this change was for my mom's convenience is absurd. My mom would have done anything for me. Our philosophy with treatment was to maintain my 'normal' life as much as possible. As for me getting psychosocial support at the hospital, after being scolded and humiliated by doctor and nurse alike I did not feel any loyalty to the clinic past the point of those who had helped me. Perhaps there is something endemically wrong at that clinic—however, my job as a 17-year-old sick patient was not to deal with that or put up with it. The move saved my treatment psychosocially. I also felt much more comfortable in the local clinic.

almost looked forward to visits to this clinic. The nurses were encouraging, supportive, often admiring of the way that Lauren was handling her treatments. They joked with her, told her stories of their pets and families, and treated her as a person who had a whole life—into which the treatment was to be fit as much as possible. There were no volunteers, no specialists (save the pediatrician), no rotating interns or residents, pharmacists, physiotherapists, or nutritionists. The social worker dropped in periodically and became, almost instantly, another source of support and encouragement.[4] We were free to call her to make additional, even regular appointments, if need be. If not, we knew she was available. At the time, there was a support group for parents, too. It met infrequently, about once per month in the hospital, and seemed to have a focus on providing information. I remember one evening talk was advertised as related to learning issues. I was never interested enough in leaving Lauren during the first year to go out for an educational event. I preferred to read and talk to individual friends and family at that time. But there were these possibilities for support—the social worker and the parent support group—if I had felt the desire.

For the first 10 months or so we visited the university-based medical centre every three weeks or so because this is where the adriamyecin was to be measured and poured into the portable pump that, as I have said, Lauren wore every three weeks for 48 hours. The scheduled three-week cycle, of course, was a mirage. To avoid an unnecessary drive the nurses at the local hospital suggested that Lauren have her blood tests in town, the day before the scheduled visit to the clinic. They also told us that this was their normal procedure. Children who needed treatment at the major medical centres, if their blood counts were high enough, were all encouraged to have their blood tests done the day before the appointment to save themselves the drive if the counts were too low. Then, if the counts were not high enough for treatment with the whole 'arsenal', families could eliminate the drive and have the part of the treatment that was not dependent on counts administered locally.

---

4   This social worker has since left the hospital. She is now a private therapist.

There are undoubtedly many reasons for the dramatic differences we experienced depending on whether the treatment was at the teaching hospital or the local one. It could have been the personalities of the nurses and doctors. It could have been their different moral, ethical, spiritual, and religious orientations. It could have been the relative size of the two clinics. It could have been the interpersonal 'chemistry'. It could have been the differential vulnerability to cut-backs experienced by the two locales. It could have been medical overspecialization. Indeed, it could have been the effect on the patient (and indirectly, on the patient's family) of being part of a research study, where perhaps the individual participant may tend to be seen more as a collection of data than as a unique human patient. Or . . .

I am not sure. But I do know that the difference in how we experienced the two locations was akin to the difference between night and day. And day was infinitely better. The suffering engendered by treatment at the local clinic was for the most part physical. It was the result of the disease and its treatment. The suffering at the big clinic was psychosocial, interpersonal, and emotional as well as medical.[5] An outline of the problems we encountered at the big city hospital clinic is provided in Table 4.

We always returned home from the big clinic at the hospital exhausted. There are some obvious reasons. We had to get up early to get down to the clinic for 8:30 a.m. or so to have Lauren's blood taken for testing, and Lauren, after all, was undergoing treatment for a serious, life-threatening disease. I was her 'worried', 'anxious' mother who increasingly feared clinic visits. The day was often fairly long by the time we were able to arrive back at our house— it was usually mid- to late afternoon. Some parts of this experience were probably unavoidable in the circumstances and these had little to do with the organization, structure, or culture of the clinic.

---

5   One clinic I entered with fear and dread, anticipating long waits, rejection, feeling ignored. The other I miss going to now that my clinic visits have been reduced. My nurses, locally, became two of the people I most consistently saw for a part of my illness, for if I was too sick for going out or school, I still needed to go to get chemo or blood taken. I, too, don't know why there is such a difference in the clinics. I pray that some healing can happen at the teaching hospital so that the future there is easier for everyone involved.

Table 4
Sources of Alienation at the Pediatric Out-patient Clinic of the Big City Hospital

Time	Order of treatment always unclear to us.
Space	No privacy for most treatments and most of the visit.
Information	Different doctors and different nurses gave us different and often conflicting and contradictory information.
Hygiene	Frequently there were children and family members with obvious colds in the clinic. The basket of cookies, open to well and ill alike for picking, is one symbol of what we thought of as unhygienic practices. Often Lauren, and undoubtedly others, was neutropenic while at the clinic, and these sanitary lapses seemed incautious if not frightening.
Noise	Usually the television was on; sometimes a video. This was never our choice. I wonder whose it was.
Changing Faces	From visit to visit the nurses on duty could differ, as could the doctor. Usually, Lauren was examined by a resident. The faces of the residents changed frequently, as did their strategies of history-taking and physical exams.

Some aspects of the clinic, however, oppress the patients and their parents.

What do we, all of us, need to feel in control? First and foremost we probably need private space in which we can do as we choose, when we choose—sleep, eat, read. Second, we need to have a sense of the organization of our time. We live by calendars and clocks. Clocks approximate the passing of a twelve-hour period. They are often digital. Time is always on the move. It is moving ahead. It is not 'about noon'. Now it is 12:02, 12:03, 12:04. It is exact. In modern North American society time is efficiency, time is money, and money is the basis for getting ahead in the world. Being in control of time is a fundamental cultural value.

People who are known to be in different places in the social structure—men as compared to women, working class as compared to middle or upper class, those of different cultural and ethnic backgrounds—have different relationships to space and time. The poor do not live in large mansions. They are not able to decide what to do with their time—at work they are more likely to punch clocks, to be paid by the hour, and to do what the boss wants. In the clinic, too, people lack control over their space and over their time.

The clinic organization engenders a similar oppression: it does not make appointments. People are supposed to be taken in the sequence in which they arrive and sign in with the receptionist at the desk. But treatments vary in many ways, including the length of time they take, which and how many personnel they include, what needs to be done in preparation, the severity of illness, a change in prognosis. These and other factors affect clinic treatments. The socializing associated with treatment varies, too. Bone marrow aspiration and lumbar puncture, for example, are infrequent but routine treatments in children with leukemia. Together they can be very time-consuming. They require the ministrations of the physician. At the teaching hospital clinic they also usually included two nurses and often a visiting doctor, a resident, or an intern as observer. Organizing all of these people to be available at one time would have been complex. It would usually be done (perhaps always) at the end of the clinic time when a doctor and two nurses could be spared at one time. The procedures usually took half an hour to an hour, and then afterwards Lauren was to be flat on her back on the hospital bed for as least one more hour. The longer she lay flat the less likely she was to suffer from a headache as a result of the lumbar puncture.

The pre-eminent treatments were the lumbar puncture and bone marrow aspiration. These were the occasions upon which all of the best medical and nursing feet were put forward. The healthcare team tried to joke, to be interesting, and to be interested in Lauren. For a few minutes while the physicians dug into the bone to retrieve some bone marrow the nurses treated Lauren compassionately and as a whole person, not just a diseased body.

On a more routine basis, however, clinic visits were exercises in anomie and powerlessness. They were anomic because we never knew what the norms or rules were, and sometimes we thought we knew but then they changed on us unexpectedly. Initially we were told that Lauren would come to the clinic every week, plan to arrive about 10 and be finished by about noon, that every three weeks she would have a series of treatments and every week other but fewer treatments. We were told that she would have her own nurse with whom she would develop a relationship of trust and warmth. None of these expectations was met.

What did happen? The first stop, once at the hospital, was the hematology lab, where Lauren would have her finger poked for blood. The blood would then be analysed and the data sent upstairs to the clinic by computer so that treatment could be planned and the drugs mixed and administered. Then we would go upstairs and wait in the waiting room outside the clinic—or eventually inside the clinic. No matter when we arrived we were essentially always the last to leave. That wasn't because we were talking to the doctor. In fact, that was another deviation from what we expected. Every three weeks Lauren was to have a physical check-up. Usually this was done by one of a parade of different residents, periodically by one of the staff doctors. The check-ups were generally very short and varied from doctor to doctor.[6] All of the staff doctors were quite different. One, for example, was warm, supportive, and caring. He always asked how Lauren (the person) was. He chatted about her interests in debating, her plans for the future, and the like. Another doctor was cold, distant, critical, and threatening. We always preferred the first doctor. But the doctors took turns. And even then, their turn-taking was infrequent because most of the time Lauren was seen by a resident. We could have coped with the taking of turns by the staff doctors and the rotating residents more easily had we known when to expect whom at the clinic, whom to prepare for on any given day.

Anomie was also perpetuated by the high density in the clinic waiting room. Not only were there all the children and their parents, even friends and other family members at times, but there was also a panoply of others—volunteers, child-life workers, social work-

---

6 I should have expected rotating doctors because we were at a teaching hospital. However, when it was only once every three weeks I thought consistency would have been more possible. The fact that a different doctor looked at my body virtually every visit leads me to question whether or not any continuity could have been achieved. My body is not the same as any other, but it does have its own pattern that changes throughout time. If one doctor saw me more consistently (as was the case once I switched to our local hospital) I would also have more confidence in discussing illnesses with her/him. As it was, my treatment at the teaching hospital lacked consistency.

ers, physiotherapists, pharmacists. We had been warned that the main thing that we had to be wary about was infections. When Lauren's counts were low she had very few white blood cells to fight a viral or bacterial infection. When children and parents, some coughing, others vomiting, waited with us in the waiting room, with the open basket of cookies on the table ready to receive germs from all takers, old magazines littering the tables, and various professionals appearing to be in varying states of health, it was difficult to imagine that the concern with infection was taken very seriously.

Stress is another term that could be used to describe our experiences, especially in the clinic. According to Lazarus (1966), whether or not an event becomes a stressor depends on personal and situational characteristics, including: (1) the degree of uncertainty, (2) the degree of loss of control, (3) the amount of threat to self esteem, and (4) the extent of the negative feelings associated. All of these have been found to be sources of stress for families whose children have received a cancer diagnosis (Van Dongen-Melman et al., 1986).

All of these characterized our visits to the university-based clinic. We were never sure whether or not Lauren would receive her planned treatments; how long we would have to wait, where we were in order, what doctor or resident or nurse would see and treat Lauren. We didn't seem to have any control over any of the above sources of uncertainty, nor did we have any sense of control over personal space.[7] 'Self-esteem is related to the image an individual has about his or her body, psychological state, and social functioning' (ibid., 150). The lack of control and uncertainty, coupled with the unpredictable and angry outbursts from the healthcare providers and, for the most part, their only superficial interest

---

[7] I remember most clinic visits as being long, tiring, and sickening. Often I would end up lying on one of my parent's laps out in the main waiting room, where patients and parents for several different clinics waited. I would feel nauseated. The noise and fluorescent lighting were sources of aggravation. Finally, I would be called in, to wait inside the cancer clinic. In the clinic the television was continuously on, showing either children's cartoons or a talk show for one of the parents. All conversations and medical interactions could be overheard and seen. The clinic had a cheerful front, however, with bald, chubby-faced kids getting orange, pink, and yellow drugs pumped into their arms.

in Lauren's life, could hardly have been designed more effectively if the intention had been to diminish and threaten Lauren's self-esteem and my confidence in my ability to ease Lauren's way as much as possible.

I have seldom in my life had to work harder at emotion management than I did in the clinic (Hochschild, 1979, 1983). My emotion-work was focused on being pleasant with the staff, trying to protect Lauren from the unpredictable assaults, and trying to look like a good mother. This emotion work was associated with the negative feeling that had developed with the clinic staff from our very first visit, when the information about the infusion of adriamyecin given by the nurse in the hospital was contradicted by the doctor, and continued from interpersonal problem to problem up until the end of treatment. Yes, the clinic was associated with negative feelings.[8] It was a major source of stress.

One of the most troublesome aspects of the available research on family coping with childhood cancer is that it tends to suggest a truncated model of stress causation and reduction. In my experience, the most important sources of stress were the medical system and the health-care providers. Dealing with these sources is, I think, much more productive than dealing with the aftermath. However, by and large the literature ignores the potential of the health-care system to cause suffering.[9] Instead, the tendency is to pathologize the family. It is as if families whose children have cancer are somehow inadequate in their functioning, inevitably traumatized and compromised by the cancer diagnosis, and comprised of psychologically inadequate mothers, fathers, and siblings.

---

8   Now in health and returning to that clinic, I find it is hard to remember that this used to be a normal part of my life. That is where I spent many days ill, just like the remaining and new patients do. Re-entering the clinic makes me both physically sick and brings tears to my eyes. Despite all the improvements in treatment there is no getting around the fact that what is happening to these kids is completely unnatural. They should be outside running around in the sun, not watching Free Willy for the fourteenth time.

9   I do not blame any particular individual for the sometimes hurtful treatment I received. However, whatever pressures the clinic was/is under created a mess of contradictory advice and recommendations for treatment. The stress and unease that this created made the clinic (and some of those associated with it) unpleasant.

Van Dongen-Melman et al. (1986) studied families in order to describe the various ways that families whose children have cancer go about coping with the stress. These include seeking information, seeking support and comfort, causal attribution, changing the situation, and, finally, using denial and avoidance. If pervasive uncertainty is a fundamental aspect of living with a serious or chronic condition over time, then seeking information, it seems to follow, would be one means of attempting to alleviate this uncertainty. Seeking comfort and support seems a useful response in two ways. In the first place, comfort and positive social support are self-evidently beneficial. In addition, however, a growing body of research documents the benefits of positive social support for quality of life and even for the length of survival after a cancer diagnosis and, indeed, in many other situations of personal health crisis (Horowitz, 1998). Finding a cause, or understanding potential causes, of a disease serves to reduce anxiety by re-establishing the sense that the world is, after all, predictable and logical. Changing the situation is another useful strategy at times. Denial and avoidance are sometimes of great benefit because they allow at least temporary relief from fear, anger, anxiety, or other negative emotions. Two other strategies suggested by Van Dongen-Melman et al. (1986) are not considered to be common. These are impulsive actions (e.g., emotional outbursts) and cognitive restructuring.

In another example, Kazak and Nachman (1991: 462) begin their review article, 'Family Research on Childhood Chronic Illness: Pediatric Oncology as an Example', with the following typical assumption: 'having a child with cancer is one of the most stressful experiences that a family can have.' Rolland (1984, 1987) outlined four dimensions of illness—onset, course, outcome, and degree of incapacitation—that are presumed to affect the family differently. Barbarin, Hughes, and Chesler (1985) describe eight coping strategies used by parents, three problem-focused (information-seeking, problem-solving, help-seeking) and five emotion-focused (acceptance, optimism, maintenance of emotional balance, denial, and religion). Kupst and her colleagues (1982) did a prospective study of family coping with and adaptation to childhood cancer and found the adjustment, as measured by a combination of self-report and semi-structured interviews, was related to social support, marital satisfaction, fewer concurrent stressors, and open communication. This research also notes that the stress is highest during the first year after diagnosis. Fife et al. (1987) found that parental anxiety declined over the year, as did involvement with outside activities. Over the period of treatment, which is generally two to three years, there may be other stressors in regard to to leukemia (Kalnins, Churchill, and Terry, 1980).

What does the research literature say about 'coping' with the problems raised in this chapter and in the chapter describing our in-patient experiences? What do we know about how people who use the health-care system experience that system? What do we know about the ways in which people in the system experience cut-backs to the system? On all accounts, not much! Most of the research literature in the area of coping with childhood cancer begins with the assumption that the childhood cancer causes the stress, and thus the subsequent coping and adjustment strategies. Childhood cancer is assumed to be the most difficult illness a family might have to endure, as evidenced by the many charitable foundations established for young cancer patients (see Chapter 11 and Appendix). This assumption, however, is not made on the basis of empirical evidence. Were it, studies of representative samples of the population would have had to have observed and/or asked 'families' how stressful they found their experience to be with all or some of numerous other problems, such as those related to chronic physical and mental health, for instance, cystic fibrosis and childhood schizophrenia, with acute episodes such as fatal or near-fatal car accidents, and with delinquency such as stealing or assaulting others. With a few exceptions (see, for example, Birenbaum, 1990) this has not been done. I do not want to diminish the suffering that is a part of the experience of a family whose child has cancer, but I do not think that the diagnosis is uniquely able to cause stress. To focus on families in this particular situation and on their adaptation, when it is based on this assumption, is problematic. It is a reflection of the stigma associated with the disease in the minds of the researchers rather than the unique consequences of this particular illness.

The assumption that this is the most stressful family experience may, in fact, exacerbate the suffering because if medical personnel think that this is the case, they may treat the family as particularly 'pitiful' and increase the degree of isolation they might feel (Stern and Arenson, 1989; Stern et al., 1991). It is perhaps a case in which the surveillance by researchers of a particular human occasion problematizes and increases the stigma and indeed may consequently increase the suffering of people in the situation.

To my mind, the most important issues to be studied relating to family coping have to do with the challenges posed by the health-care system: it is one thing to have a child with cancer, it is another to have to deal with the inadequacies and contradictions of the health-care system that I have described. Nevertheless, an enormous literature within the discipline of social psychology describes and analyses family coping with childhood cancer as if the source of stress has to do with the diagnosis, not the treatment. Families whose children have cancer are assumed to be pathological. Three common presuppositions follow:

> 'The literature strongly indicates that families experience serious difficulties and are a population at risk of developing psychosocial problems' (Van Dongen-Melman et al., 1986: 145).
>
> Parents' coping styles are psychologically diagnosable: 'Parents use of denial to ward off their own fear resulted in a decrease in anxiety but also limited perception of the needs of the other family members' (ibid., 159).
>
> Parents' initial response to the diagnosis can be 'characterized as a state of shock that may last for several weeks. Severe neurotic symptoms can easily develop during this phase. Anxiety and depression may occur in up to 50% of parents' (ibid.).

Another researcher followed the course of parental adjustment to find that 12–18 months after the initial period of treatment 28 per cent of the mothers of leukemic children were depressed and anxious to a morbid degree (Maguire, 1983). In addition, the stress of 'coping with childhood cancer may cause health problems, alcohol abuse, social isolation, sexual and marital difficulties' (Van Dongen-Melman et al., 1986; 159). Again, because researchers have assumed psychopathology in parents whose children had cancer, we find a psychiatric inventory applied to parents who were, indeed, discovered to have two kinds of psychopathology: 'Thirteen of the 18 suffered symptoms of anxiety outside the normal range: of these 13, six had moderate or severe symptoms which warranted further attention. A group of six parents showed marked communication difficulty with staff, friends and their own spouses' (Hughes and Lieberman, 1990: 53).

Other studies, however, have not assumed or looked for pathology in the parents. One such study of 33 families asked the families to define and describe the issues that were important to them in their responses to cancer in their children (Martinson and Cohen, 1988). In this case the parental perceptions were described, not diagnosed. Fifteen themes emerged from the interviews.

1. Parents were unprepared for the diagnosis.
2. They initially relinquished control over the management of the disease.
3. Their needs for information were initially satisfied.
4. They developed stategies for managing probabilistic information.
5. They had fears about bringing the child home from the hospital.
6. They needed to normalize family life.
7. They became dependent on the medical center for care.
8. They reclaimed control over the management of the disease.
9. They feared that the patient's disease would recur.
10. They became increasingly dissatisfied with the quality and quantity of the information they were given as death approached.
11. They experienced a sense of relief when the child died.
12. They used symbols and rituals to cope with illness and death.
13. They found that anniversaries of stressful times were especially difficult.
14. They feared that a sibling might develop cancer.
15. They had difficulty managing the response of siblings. (Ibid., 83)

A somewhat unusual article begins with the assertion that childhood cancer is one of the most stressful situations a family can experience, but then goes on to note that 'the medical staff can help exacerbate or mediate such stress and has a major impact on the parents' views about the quality of care they and their children receive' (Lozowski et al., 1993: 64). Significantly, at least one of the authors of this study is also a parent whose daughter had cancer as a child. Possibly this 'subjective' vantage point helped him point the way to seeing that family functioning is not endogenous to the uniqueness of the disease but also is affected by such exogenous factors as medical care. These researchers found that parents' reports of intervention for improvement in the care of their children were 'commonplace'.

Birenbaum is another researcher who has not assumed that childhood cancer is uniquely the most stressful situation faced by a family. Using the CHIP scale (a standardized measure called Coping Health Inventory for Parents), she compared the results of answers given by 45 parents of children with cancer to those from parents who had children with different diagnoses. With respect to the subscales studied, i.e., medical communication, family integration and support, esteem, and stability, 'parents' coping was similar to other samples of families with childhood chronic illness' (Birenbaum, 1990: 31).

Some studies try to show that how parents handle their children's disease affects the long-term psychosocial adjustment of the children, as well as their own future lives. 'Although other studies have demonstrated the importance of parental reactions to the process of adjusting to childhood cancer, the present study emphasized the importance of these variables, even years after successful treatment' (Overholser and Fritz, 1990: 81).

I am not the only family member who has felt her (or his) role diminished and her intentions demeaned by a health-care providers and health policy. Michael Klein, whose wife, Bonnie Klein, a renowned Canadian film-maker had two strokes and who wrote the story of her illness and recovery in *Slow Dance: A Story of Stroke, Love and Disability*, described his own experience in the *Canadian Medical Association Journal*. Klein, a physician, spent a great deal of time in the hospital with his wife during a period of six months:

> during the more than 6 months in 3 hospitals, I found Bonnie's care less than optimal on many occasions. The medical and nursing staff varied in their response to these discoveries. At times they were grateful for my intervention and responded with corrective measures. On other occasions some were angry and suggested that I was over-involved and meddlesome (Klein, 1997: 55).

He describes a number of such occasions, some life-threatening and others causing his wife extreme suffering. He intervened repeatedly and, even though his interventions undoubtedly helped and even saved his wife, he was frequently rebuked and chastised by his colleagues. His plea is that family members be integrated into the care of their loved ones. As he says:

> the irony is that anyone who has worked in an institution knows that mistakes are inevitable. People and machines are fallible, and in the end we need all the help we can get. Family members, physicians or not, need to be integrated into the care of their loved one. Their ideas must not be trivialized, their concerns demeaned. (Ibid.)

This insight from a doctor whose wife was critically ill has some relevance to our situation and points to a lack in the research literature. The literature on families with children who have cancer is almost devoid of attention to mistakes, inadequacies, and problems in the health-care system or to the possible positive role that parents and loved ones might provide.

Questions such as the following need to be asked and answers to them sought. Why did we experience anger, rigidity, sneering, and what we thought of as sexism from one doctor in the clinic, on the one hand, and warmth, encouragement, compassion, and some seeming befuddlement from another clinic doctor? I calibrated on an extremely fine scale every reaction of each doctor. I wanted clear, precise information based on state-of-the-art research; ability to answer questions, to find the answers to questions, or to inform us when questions were unanswered given the available scientific findings; and respect and compassion towards my daughter and myself. I know that I expected a lot, and my every sense was attuned to measuring whether or not, and to what extent, the doctors met my expectations. I suspect that my highly sensitized observation and evaluation of the doctors was exacerbated by the gravity of the illness. I can't remember a relationship in which I have been so very highly strung—so, for my part, I must admit that my easygoing, forgiving, optimistic side was totally in abeyance. I was a mother bear fervently trying to protect her cub, ever attentive to the slightest whiff of danger—whether emotional, mental, or physical. These were the sources of the emotion-work in which I was constantly engaged.

What could explain the part of my experience that was generated by the physicians? We could probably all agree that the ideal in a situation such as this is that the doctors are seen as minimizing stress by offering compassion and clear, consistent information. These ideals were not met. Not only were these ideals unmet, their causes or political solutions are not adequately understood by health researchers, policy-makers, or health-care providers.

Chapter 7

Back to Normal?

Lauren had hoped that her lifeline would be going back to school. It was to be her key to normality and selfhood. She was in grade 12. She had one OAC in Latin from a previous year and she had a minimum of five more to do before going to university. She had been planning to finish high school over two more years so that she would have lots of choices in the future. By taking a full two years she would have been able to take more of the courses that she wanted to take. It would also mean that her alternatives for university were broadened. Just before she was diagnosed she had made the decision to go on to university the next year and to take six OACs, the required number and no more. Then, during the initial remission induction, she debated about whether she would be able to do all six courses. It very quickly became apparent that one of her courses, biology, would be impossible to continue because of the required daily lab exercises and reports. She was not going to be able to go to school every day. That left three courses to continue with in the first term—film studies, creative writing, and French.[1]

They could not have been better courses to be taking right then. She was able to watch movies in the hospital and as she was recuperating at home. The assignment in her creative writing course was a magazine. It was to be a group project. The group that she was a part of sent a note and said that they would be happy to have her continue in the group and do whatever she could. But Lauren eventually decided that she would prefer to do her own

---

[1] I thought at the beginning that I would be able to return to my classes. How wrong a perception this turned out to be. But I had a supportive school behind me. The teachers helped me and modified programs. My French teacher brought laughter with his weekly teachings and this was wonderful.

assignment independently since she didn't know if she would be able to do her fair share of the work in the group context. Thus, she typed up a proposal for a magazine for teens with cancer. Her teacher approved her topic. Her French literature course involved reading and essay writing. Again, she thought she would be able to do this in the hospital and at home while she was recuperating. Her high school assigned a home-school teacher, who coincidentally was her French teacher. He helpfully carried messages back and forth from Lauren to the film studies and creative writing teachers.

Lauren was not able to go back to school at all the first term. She was diagnosed in mid-October and out of the hospital in mid-

> **Openers**
>
> Hello! This magazine is a look at some of the issues with which I as a teen with leukemia am dealing. At the time of this publication I've been diagnosed for a little over three months. The writing in this magazine comes from my experiences and new knowledge throughout these three months.
>
> I have shifted from the newness of having the disease and getting a diagnosis to the reality of living with the disease. This has not been an easy experience. I will be living with the disease for the next two years. Sometimes, it is not a good place to be. However, it will get better. I have had some very scary, devastating moments as well as some times of joy. Lots of people have tried to tell me about my disease and most of the time I have asked them to stop. Some information has not been good for me to hear and that was hard. This magazine may have some things in it that you associate with, or it may not.
>
> Writing this magazine is partly a way of showing that I can do it. It is partly to get information for myself. Finally, it is a way of putting the last months into a little more perspective.
>
> Really, it is what I could have used in the first three months of my illness. . . .
>
> From Lauren's magazine for teen cancer patients, *Healing Hands, Fighting Fists* (Spring 1996).

November but undergoing daily radiation until the beginning of December. By then there were just a few weeks until Christmas vacation, and we suspected lots of colds and flu would be around the school. Lauren's counts were very low; she was very vulnerable to infection, and felt quite sick and tired. Again, after Christmas in early January, she did not return to school because there was just a part of a week of school before exams. The possibility of infection weighed against the amount of instruction that Lauren would miss. She continued to feel quite ill and fatigued, as well, and so she decided to stay at home.

In the middle of January, she had a fever and had to be hospitalized for a two-week period in order to be on intravenous antibiotics and, in fact, missed the first few days of the second term. But as soon she was able to start back she did so, with one class a day. She had previously planned a seminar course in French with her teacher and two other students. This was to be a study of the theatre of the absurd. The course involved just three meetings with the group and teacher and the writing of a play (in French) in the absurd tradition. During the second term she continued to complete all the assignments for the first term that she had yet to hand in, as well as the work for the second term courses.

The first day that Lauren went back to class she felt really weak and sick. I drove her to the door, walked her to her classroom, and carried in a special folding chair, situated by the door for her to sink comfortably into and so that she would be near the door in case she had to leave quickly because of nausea, exhaustion, or some other unnamed calamity.[2] This class was a bit more than an hour long. I waited in the parking lot, right outside the school door, in case she needed help. She managed to stay in class. The next day I

---

2 This first day going back was hard. All the people I wanted to see I didn't due to class times and my tiredness. The others in my class were acquaintances, but none were very good friends. As I walked up the stairs, slowly, lifting my legs by hand, my mom standing beside me, I remember people staring. It was difficult because these people, just months before, had known me as energetic, involved, and outgoing. Now I was a stooping, slow, hat-bedecked stranger. Over time, especially once my mom wasn't there and people grew used to my new appearance, it was easier. However, for the remainder of my high school days I was sick.

parked the car and waited in the school library. This continued for about one week. After this I went home, which was about five minutes by car, and sat working by the phone at my desk. Lauren never called to come home early. I, however, was still on guard. I always waited by the phone and if someone called I quickly ended the conversation with a promise to call back at a later time.

I dropped her off at a back door to the school. This minimized her walk through the bustling, pushing, and shoving that to me, in my new fear, characterized the hallways. She had to climb a few stairs into the school, which for her at this time was a miraculous feat. But she did it up one step at a time, with her backpack full of books, writing material, and lunch! On the days that she went to school, probably half of the possible days, she managed to stay for the whole time. Almost always, she took a few minutes after class to socialize with her friends and then called when she was ready to go home. She usually emerged from the school with her backpack slung across her shoulder and her boyfriend Michael at her side.

Most often she would have some food after school and we would go immediately to an aquatics class at a local pool. She loved this exercise because it was gentle, warm, and comforting; she rarely missed a class. Once in a while I would go with her, but I mostly sat and watched her, through the window, the only young person within a small group of elderly, grey-haired women.[3]

Her high school teachers all were marvelous. The teacher in the one class that she actually attended had agreed to let Lauren come when she could, to write tests at school or at home, and to hand in work as she was able. He gave us his home number so that we could keep in touch if Lauren needed notes, assignments, films, or anything else when she had to miss school. He did not deduct any marks for missed classes and was absolutely flexible about her

---

[3] One of the major turning points in my physical recovery was the first time I entered the local hot pool. My mom said that watching me was as simple as between not smiling (pre-pool) and smiling. At first, all my energy was diverted into putting on my swimming suit and getting into the pool. Later I was able to start the 'elderly' aquatics. Currently, I participate in my university aquatics programs. In fact, it thrills me to be stronger than some of my classmates in push-ups or lunges. Me, strong again? Yes, and it is wonderful!

schedule. The one thing that she planned a few months ahead, and was able to carry off, was a seminar for this teacher, of about one hour, in front of the class. By the time May came around and her day of presentation arrived, she was able to sit in front of this class on a stool for the whole hour and talk to the group. Sitting up and concentrating while keeping the attention of the class was, to me, an awesome accomplishment. To soften and sweeten up the class she began by handing around tins of Chinese cookies and candies. Afterwards, she, Jess, and I went out to lunch at one of her favourite places to celebrate.

At first, when she returned to school she said some of the teachers avoided her, while others didn't seem to know what to say to her. I called the principal and asked if he thought it would be a good idea for me to give a talk about Lauren and her disease and treatment to a meeting of the teachers. He did, and arranged for me to have five minutes of the agenda at a meeting where virtually all of the teachers were in attendance. I told the teachers that she was going to get better, that she was already in remission, and that they would notice that she felt better some days than others and that this was due to the cycle of treatment rather than the disease. I explained that the reason she looked so ill was not the disease but the treatment. The teachers seemed to respond well and from then on were friendly with Lauren. We believed that they hadn't known what to say. The idea that one of their students, and one who was well known to most, if not all of the teachers, because of her active involvement in the school as president of various clubs, was so seriously ill must have been devastating for them.

As one of the teachers later said, when asked by a friend (and after the teacher agreed to be quoted): 'Initially, there was a lot of worry and concern among the teachers. You always think the worst—you're programmed to think that's the end. Initially the reaction was oh-oh. This is really tragic. Then as Juanne mentioned at the staff meeting—the information was very important to have. She told us there's all kinds of options here. It was important for us to have that information, and for Lauren to know that information. You never think of it striking someone who's a really popular student.'

The social life of her friends and classmates continued. They had parties, went to shows, concerts, and just 'out' to hang around. At school the things that Lauren had been involved in continued. Student council, debating, federal-provincial simulation, the environment club, the gender relations club, the newspaper, and all of the other informal social and extracurricular activities: they all continued but Lauren could not keep up with them. She couldn't go to parties because she often felt too sick or too tired from her chemotherapy treatments or because her counts were too low and she was excessively vulnerable to picking up the germs and bacteria that populate all of us at intervals.

Lauren's social life consisted of visits from her friends, usually one at a time, and watching movies on video.[4] We watched more movies in those months than before or since. One other diversion, a horrifyingly banal and boring ritual, was to watch whatever was on television from about four o'clock until seven or eight, with some time to try to eat some food. On the weekends Jess often returned home from university to visit and several times a week friends and family dropped by with muffins or flowers or candles or other wonderful surprises.

Lauren and I had similar but different experiences regarding the reactions of our friends to the diagnosis and to living with the treatments over time. I guess the first interesting thing to me was how secondary my friends became as compared to the immediacy and the urgency of what was going on with Lauren and the reactions of my immediate family. I didn't have the energy to call to let them know. I wasn't even thinking of them or how they might be doing for the first few months or more. Instead, my focus was on Lauren, then her sister, and then my mother, my sister, and my brother. Day after day my sister Cindy came to the hospital to visit, always bringing something special with her like home-made chocolate chip banana muffins. It was this sister who finally got me to eat after at least a week during which I couldn't even think about food,

---

4   This ritual became one of my favourites. Although it was numbing and dull, Mom and I would do it basically every night, cuddling on the couch. It was a time when I didn't need to do anything or be anyone except myself. These were comforting hours. I usually didn't feel ill then.

when she brought me a fresh fruit salad.

My mom was on alert because, on that Thanksgiving visit just prior to the diagnosis, she had inspected under Lauren's eyes and her fingernails and was sure that there was something wrong with her blood because she was so pale. As I was growing up she was vigilant about health. My reaction to this had been to more or less ignore ill health except insofar as I could act preventively. My daughters and I were fairly conscientious about our diet, exercise, sleep, and the like. But I had never been particularly somatically, or bodily, focused. In fact, I rarely went to the doctor. I had gone during my pregnancies and then just once or twice in the 20 or so intervening years. Neither had I taken the children to the doctor frequently—except for camp check-ups, serious recurrent earaches, and two cases of pneumonia. My orientation had always been that the body wants to be healthy—and needs good food, exercise, and rest to stay healthy. But I hadn't looked for symptoms of illness or gone to the doctor for myself or the children for routine annual visits or whenever a flu or cold had struck. My mother's (hyper)vigilance had become my insouciance. As I have said earlier, the contemporary focus on health promotion and disease prevention provided a legitimation for my approach to health.

In any case, Mom's reaction was to panic and bake. We had said, knowing that she would want to know what she could do, that she could make butter tarts. She and her sisters—there were five sisters still alive then—were all famous in the family for their baking and cooking. Butter tarts were among the family favourites. My brother brought my mom down to the hospital laden with tarts and she came and stood at the door with a mask on. Her other reactions were shielded from me as much as possible by my brother and sister who, thankfully calmed her and answered her questions. After we were settled at home, about a month and a half after diagnosis, I started to call my mother fairly regularly. I always said (as I recall) that Lauren was okay, that she was perhaps feeling a bit sick today but was definitely on the road to recovery. I knew I didn't want to have to deal with her anxiety as well as my own and for the most part the strategy worked that we decided upon early, which depended on my brother and sister taking care of Mom.

Later on, after a few months, Mom would call on days when Lauren was to have gone to have treatment. Often, of course, treatment was postponed. She would question whether Lauren had received treatment. We always said yes, because she did receive L'asparagenese every week, even though Lauren was not receiving the treatment she was supposed to receive, and my mother would respond positively to this information. I felt the potential of being judged a failure as a mother, that she was checking up on me. Every time this happened it was, I expect, my mother's anxiety that forced her to ask questions, her need to hear the positive, the correct answer all the time. For my mother and her sisters, childhood cancer brought back many fears and heartbreaks. Lauren and I needed to maintain strategies to distance ourselves from the additional anxiety that this history engendered and, for the most part, we succeeded. In any case, telling and managing my mom was dealt with by my sister and brother. What had to be done with Lauren had to be done. Jess was always a source of support, compassion, and understanding.

I was 'strong' enough in the little context of my immediate family—Lauren and Jess, Cindy and Rich—but I was not thinking of people outside of this little group yet. I was staying with Lauren full-time. Even when I went to the washroom or for a shower I rushed. A shower was a three-minute affair. I needed to be with Lauren to try to protect her. In the hospital, taking care of Lauren was my only concern—just being with her, helping her ask questions of the doctors and nurses, holding her hand, cooling her with a wet cloth when necessary, helping to change the sheets when they were soaked, helping her and her IV pole to the bathroom, rubbing her back, and standing guard against medical mistakes or mischance. No matter how kind or competent each individual professional was, I knew Lauren better and loved her more than each one of the staff. Protecting her from too many visits, even from staff, by posting a note on the door; asking people to leave when their presence was simply 'too much'; getting popsicles and such from the fridge; trying to get one of the VCRs (before we brought our own in) and find suitable videos—these were among my many mundane tasks and were my complete focus. Then, when we were home I had a more regular routine to manage. Lauren needed help with showering, sometimes with dressing and choosing clothes. I generally prepared food, kept the house clean (reasonably), sat with Lauren to watch videos, talked with her about her courses, drove her to school, aquatics, and so on. In any case, my focus and most of my time were taken up with the routines involved in helping a sick person.

A couple of weeks after Lauren's diagnosis my sister had called my office and several of my closest friends. I didn't want to leave Lauren and I was too upset to be far enough away from her to have an independent conversation about how I felt. I guess I was too devastated to begin to acknowledge it at all. When we were in the hospital during the first month I got word that someone had broken into our house and taken some things. I had to go home to investigate and then report this to the police and insurance company. I went home one Sunday morning and my brother came with me to change the locks. While in town I took a few minutes to go to my office to get some mail. I needed to get hold of a manuscript for the second edition of a book on health, illness, and medicine that needed to be proofread. There, at the office, I ran into one of my 'bosses'. He had heard and said how ironic it was that I was studying the politicization of breast cancer and my daughter was now sick with cancer. He commiserated with me and I bravely told him not to worry, that we were doing fine and that Lauren's prognosis was excellent. Devastated or not, I could not show it to others or acknowledge it to myself.

This boss was not the only one to comment on the irony of me, a sociologist with an interest in the social dynamics of health, illness, and medicine and a special interest in the experience, social psychology, and politics of cancer, having a daughter diagnosed with the disease. I never found it easy to respond to the comment. Was I to laugh? To say, 'Yes, isn't it something'? I always felt that the comment had something of the 'it serves you right—play with fire and you'll get burned' philosophy of life. It also reminded me of the just-world hypothesis that social psychologists have used to explain a common reaction of people when friends or acquaintances suffer a serious, catastrophic, or any other unpleasant life event. The just-world hypothesis is the tendency that people have to explain the misfortune of others as somehow or other the result of actions that the others have taken.[5] It serves to distance the person who is currently or still a non-sufferer from the sufferer. It is a way for the non-sufferer to confirm for himself or herself that he/she is different from and therefore not vulnerable to the sort of catastrophe presently experienced by the others (Stahley, 1988).

I was uninterested in telling more distant friends. I belonged to a women's group—a group that I had been a member of from the time Lauren was an infant. In fact, I breast-fed her during an

> **Just World**
>
> When I got sick with leukemia different people tried to explain it in different ways. The most common was that it was unfair ... that it was a bad, horrible, and unjust occurrence. However, one person said that she wasn't surprised that I got leukemia because I work so hard.
>
> This explanation is based on the just-world hypothesis. This hypothesis is simply that everything must have a reason ... that I caused my illness by my own choices. If a person gets sick it is this person's own fault. The world is just, and people who suffer from one thing or another are therefore to blame.
>
> If you do something good you will be rewarded. If something bad happens, you must have been bad.
>
> I guess what I am learning is that this is not a just world. I don't know that everything happens for a reason. I believe that we can find reason in everything but not that things have an inherent reason.
>
> I do not deserve to suffer from cancer. No one deserves cancer.
>
> From Lauren's magazine for teen cancer patients, *Healing Hands, Fighting Fists* (Spring 1996).

---

5   One of my friends commented to Meaghan, my best friend, that she thought I was sick because of how busy I had been. That was a devastating blow. In the case of childhood leukemia, where the mean age of patients is four years old, it seems unlikely that behaviour plays much of a role.

early meeting. This group met approximately once a month. The purpose of the group had been to provide support to one another. I hadn't seen them since August. The fall had been a busy one. And now I didn't have the time or energy to explain to them what was happening.

When I reflect back on the time it seems to me that there were people who just had to know. It is hard to qualify or characterize this group otherwise, but a blueprint or program was in place, just as with our sitting arrangement when the news was broken initially. Some people had to know; for others, it simply didn't matter. This rigid patterning or closeness and distance of relationship seemed a solace somehow, a bedrock provision of security. It was as if there was a moral obligation to tell certain people and to make sure that others knew. There were other people I really had to tell, but they lived further away or would need explanation and reassurance from me—several old friends who lived thousands of miles away, two younger women who had been almost daughters to me, and sisters to Lauren and Jess, and who had lived with us at times during their own tumultuous teen years. There were others who had to know, over time, and others who would perhaps find out as the word spread through various friendship and neighbourhood circles.

The word did spread and surprises began to happen. The most assiduous offers of help and support came, at times, from people from whom I would have least expected such help. A colleague from another department at the university, with whom I had had several dinners, hiked, and skated, wondered where I was, called around, and found out from my department secretary that I was in the hospital with one of my daughters. She called every few days and offered all kinds of university-related services as well as friendship. Some others sent wonderful baskets and bouquets of flowers and came down to visit—even if it was only possible to visit for a few minutes. Another colleague really wanted to help. She asked what she could do. She offered to come down, to bring my mail, to help with some related matters—such as applying for a sabbatical the next year. She found a home for our cat while we were in the hospital and provided food and kitty litter and made a scratching post for him.

So immediate reactions of different people surprised me. In the meantime, some of my closest friends became distant. One was busy with crises and stress in her own life. In another case the distancing was more dramatic. This friend seemed even more anxious and particular than I was. She quizzed me in detail about Lauren's diet, told me that she had read that diet was really important—at the time, Lauren could hardly keep anything down. At this time, although I was aware of the importance of good food, I was anxious to have Lauren eat some calories—any calories. It was so hard for her to eat. Her appetite was fickle and once she had eaten she often got sick. So advice about food, advice I knew already, was not helpful. Such advice, if anything, encouraged me to think about whether I ought to be feeling guilty for the choices I was making. In fact, I quickly realized that guilt was neither appropriate nor necessary. But my separation from my friend was begun. (This rift has completely healed now.) She asked a lot of questions and gave advice. Both were really hard for me at this time. I didn't have answers to any of the really important questions, and they were the only questions that I thought about at the time. Questions like: Is there anything I can to do to help Lauren to feel less nausea, less tiredness? Is there anything I can do to help her feel more optimism, pleasure, or even joy on this day, at this time? My concentration was so focused on Lauren and how she was feeling and how to keep her feeling better that the questions—about prognosis, about drugs and their effects, about alternatives, about whether she was able to receive her chemotherapy or not, about the consequences of her low count—were a bother, however well intended and sincere. I didn't want to answer other people's questions. A barrage of questions at this time seemed to heighten my anxiety. If I just knew the answers then everything would be all right, or so it seemed. Unfortunately for me, I had wanted them to tell me not to worry, that it would be all right. Instead, some wanted or needed to rely on me for that. Advice wasn't helpful either. I spent all day every day thinking about what we could do about various problems and issues that we encountered. My sense was that advice was irrelevant. Unless it had been solicited, any advice seemed to me to reflect a lack of understanding.

A big surprise was how much we valued meals as treats. The first day we arrived home from the hospital, neighbours brought us over a thermal bag with casseroles, sparkling cider, fresh fruits, and desserts. It was ready to be eaten right away—still warm from the oven. It was also freezable and had freezing instructions included. Other neighbours responded with delicious dinners, muffins, cookies, and flowers. Over the next year, another friend made soup or pasta on about a weekly basis and brought it over. Often we would come home from school, swimming or the clinic—our only outings during that first winter—to find a marvellous home-made soup in a big jar or a casserole between the front doors. Sometimes the same friend came by with flowers and talked if we had time. Others brought over pavlova, turkey and dressing, cakes, cookies, and tarts. Another friend made about a dozen frozen dinners of pastas, quiches, vegetable pies, and soups. We had a full-size freezer and so these treats were spectacular. I had no idea beforehand how much food could be appreciated. I was so busy with Lauren and so lacking in imagination for cooking that presents of food were manna from heaven. Other friends offered to sit with Lauren any time I needed or wanted to go out. I appreciated these offers, but I needed and wanted to be with her all the time so I never took anyone up on this possibility.

It would be hard to generalize from our experience to the experience of others. It would also be difficult to make suggestions for others who are wanting to offer friendship and support to someone who is going through something similar to what we were going through. I found that I did not have any expectations of help from other people, at first. So when people asked what they could do to help, I had no answers—and being asked and having to think of an answer felt like work to me. I did not even have the energy to plan for our needs beyond the moment or the day. When the food started to arrive I was absolutely stunned and very grateful. Eating and cooking had never been big issues to me. I had always been fairly flexible, though my daughters and I tended to be vegetarians. Lauren's food desires changed all the time during this period. Something that tasted good one night often did not taste good the next night, so planning ahead for Lauren seemed impossible. I often took a quick trip down to the grocery store to pick up something that Lauren fancied on the spur of the moment. In any case, for us the gifts of food were wonderful.

At the same time, it was difficult to answer when people asked, 'What can I do?' Frequently, what would have been really helpful would have been to have someone to call or go to the grocery or video store at the last moment just when we realized what we wanted. But this did not seem a reasonable request to make of anyone. Another thing that would have been helpful would have been to have an on-call psychotherapist-type person—someone who would just listen to my anxieties and fears. Often, there was no other response that I wanted. Everything that could be done was apparently being done, at least medically speaking. I also had all kinds of medical questions I couldn't ask the doctors or for which they did not have answers. For example, Lauren had to use a mouthwash four times a day, and she hated the taste. Every time she tried to take it she gagged and felt as if she was going to be sick. I called all across the country to the centres where I knew there were pediatric oncology clinics, as well as to various manufacturers, to see if there were other flavours. Ironically, while I did not get answers from any of these far-flung telephone forays, Lauren finally found a palatable flavour at the local community hospital when we finally, in the spring, had occasion to fill the prescription locally. It would have been wonderful if someone else had taken on that task and found the answer that we eventually found (or another useful answer), but that is the sort of thing that is difficult to ask someone else to do.

There were instrumental tasks like painting and moving furniture to and around the family room so that Lauren could have comfortable room for homework, relaxing, and having friends in on the first floor. A group of family members did that for us. As I search my brain for what was helpful I think that people listening, responding to requests, and taking the initiative with small or larger gifts of flowers or food were all most helpful.

It is difficult for people to know what to do and it is also difficult at a time like this to know what to ask people to do.[6] Everything has changed suddenly and drastically in the lives of the family with a child who is critically ill. All of the taken-for-granted ways of relating are challenged. It is probably inevitable that social, friendship, and family relationships are stressed and strained and that some are stronger after such a personal crisis and others are weaker. This is not because people don't care or don't want to help (in my experience, people care terribly and some are even immobilized by concern) but they simply do not know what to do. And we, as the family in the crisis, because we are living on the edge of time, from moment to moment, do not know what to ask for. Besides, we are all different in some ways. One person might find planning and cooking meals to be an escape and a chance to regain some balance. Another might cherish some time alone and appreciate the assistance of sitting with the sick child or babysitting siblings. Most everyone probably appreciates a listening, non-judgemental, and supportive ear.

One study of relationships between families of children with cancer and their friends found that while many families do manage to cope with the childhood cancer diagnosis effectively, sometimes even by enhancing family cohesion, many reported that they had difficulties in seeking help from friends. Parents expressed a number of worries about relationships with friends, including: (1) the emotional impact of the diagnosis on friends; (2) how to balance their competing needs for help and privacy; (3) maintaining the balance of give and take in the friendship; (4) sensitivity about the stigma of needing help; (5) uncertainty about the effectiveness of help; and (6) issues related, particularly among men, to overcoming sex-role barriers in regard to giving and receiving help. Unfortunately, these researchers found that such difficulties 'not only make it hard for parents to seek help and for friends to provide help, but they may cause some help to be ineffective and/or unsatisfying, and escalate parents'

---

6   I think the most important thing is perhaps the hardest, and that is to break the silence. Sympathy, empathy, hello, how are you, I love you, I miss you—all are things I needed to hear. The silence was the most difficult. The most helpful were just the simple words by phone or letter saying that people were thinking about us and praying for us.

stress' (Chesler and Barbarin, 1984: 128).

Receiving or asking for help was new territory for me. I had always been fairly self-sufficient and independent. If anything, I was the helper. We had always, as a family, made it a point to offer 'help' to others. My grandmother had died just a few years earlier at 98 years of age. During most of the lives of my daughters, when we were home on a Sunday we would visit Grandma. From the time Lauren was six years old we had been involved, first as a family and later both Jess and Lauren separately, with a local organization called Extend-A-Family. Our involvement began with a regular weekly evening spent with a girl with special cognitive and motor disabilities. We would pick her up on our way home from school. I had been on various social service boards, including the United Way and the District Health Council. From the time Lauren and Jess were little we had sent money to an international development agency in support of four children. Our sense that we were privileged and wanted to share and 'help' others was strong. So this was a very different position for us to be in, and more often than not I did not really know what would be helpful until after I had received it.

Chapter 8

Committing Complementary Care

I have long been interested in alternative and complementary medicines. In fact, I had taken my children and myself to a naturopathic doctor over the years for regular check-ups and care. I had also taken the children to allopathic doctors whenever there had been a somatic 'crisis'. When Jess was about eight she ran in a cross-country race on a very cold day and developed severe and acute asthma. For this I took her to the emergency room of the local hospital. She was admitted and we stayed overnight. When this turned to pneumonia she was prescribed an antibiotic. When Lauren was a little girl she had periodic ear infections. Again, when the pain was acute I took her to the allopathic doctor who prescribed antibiotics. This happened several times. She also had her tonsils removed because of recurring infections. When Lauren was about six she developed eczema. The dermatologist prescribed a cortisone-based cream, threatened her with death if she scratched (because it could spread all over her body and result in open bleeding sores),[1] and charged me with being a bad mother because I worked (outside of the home for money). This interaction was entirely unsatisfactory.

I started looking at books on allergy and eczema—and tried rotating diets, changing cloths, fabrics, and soaps. These attempts were unsuccessful. Lauren was never able to maintain a rotary diet. Instead, she traded her boring lunch-time pineapple juice and similar 'healthy' fare for such exciting options from friends at school as Oreo cookies. The soap changes didn't seem to make any difference. The eczema always got better in the summer and worse in the winter. Every time

---

[1] Luckily, this interaction remains forgotten to me. However, I wonder how it affects my current interactions with doctors? Do I perceive them as doomsayers forecasting my imminent death due to my own naughty actions?

a new skin cream was introduced to the market we tried it—some would give relief overnight or temporarily. Visiting the naturopath was fun—he was always willing to listen—but the eczema didn't clear up. A few years before Lauren's leukemia diagnosis I ran into an old friend one day who remarked that her migraines, which she had had for 20 years, were disappearing as a result of a 'Chinese' doctor in a nearby town. Lauren and I went to this doctor for her eczema. He said that her condition was serious—far more serious than mine—and yet he said I needed treatment for 'heart' problems. He prescribed herbal drinks, which Lauren barely tolerated even though they seemed to be working. Over time she just couldn't stand the taste.[2] I found the taste horrid but I managed to swallow the remedies in a few big gulps. These treatments worked for both of us. Chest pains that I had had ended and Lauren's skin cleared up. In any case, we were not averse to trying alternative complementary treatments.

Leukemia, I thought, was not a disease to be treated with complementary medicine.[3] I knew enough to know that the protocols of chemotherapy and radiation were quite successful and the best chance Lauren had with this desperately aggressive and life-threatening illness. However, they were also very toxic. With each drug there was a warning. The drugs could be hard on the liver, kidneys, pancreas, spleen, and heart—indeed, every organ in the body. Nausea, vomiting, malaise, and fatigue were expected side-effects of the weekly drug mixtures that Lauren was taking. In addition, radiation seemed to cause generalized suffering for a time.

What could we do? What could I do to help her with the side-effects? The clinic doctors prescribed ondonsetron for the immediate nausea and vomiting associated with the adriamyecin and the

---

2   These herbal drinks consist of boiling down large amounts of herbs and other natural ingredients into a drink. The smell alone would make me nauseated. Now, this doctor offers me pills that are not as effective as the home-brewed medicine but are swallowable.

3   I have heard of others who have gone the 'natural' route to recovery. I applaud them and their health-care givers. However, for me I was looking at a plus 80 per cent (now we know it's plus 90 per cent) recovery rate based on chemotherapy drugs. I didn't really consider an alternative. The allopathic method (which I usually had shied away from) was going to work and that is all I needed to hear.

heavy infusion of methotrexate. Every time Lauren had an infusion/injection of adriamyecin she also had a prescription of ondonsetron for 48 hours. Other than that, and the recommendation to take Tylenol and Gravol when needed, the side-effects seemed to be basically our business.

There was a sign at the clinic admonishing parents, and the admitting doctor warned us, to inform the medical staff of any other drugs, such as vitamins or herbal medicines, that a child might be taking. We had experiences with each of the two clinic doctors, however, that led us to be reluctant to explain our possible search for alternatives. When Lauren asked Dr M about itchiness, which may have been related to the antibiotic, he said, in what was a very demeaning and perhaps sexist tone, 'Well, have a bath.' When Lauren was constantly feeling nauseated we tried things like ginger teas, ginger ales, and various other folk remedies. One suggestion several people made, and that was in fact printed in a booklet of information handed out by the clinic, was a motion sickness bracelet. Lauren tried it, but it did not seem to work. Gravol, the medically prescribed alternative, made her sleepy and 'out of it'.[4] We asked Dr M if he had any suggestions. He asked what we had tried. When we mentioned the motion sickness bracelet he 'sneered', but he didn't offer any other options. When we asked another doctor about vitamin C, which we had always taken at the threat of a cold with good results, he said warmly that his wife made him take it and he guessed it would be okay. We asked how much, and he said that his wife gave him 4,000 milligrams when he was getting a cold. Clearly, these doctors were not going to be able to help us make decisions about the potential use of complementary medicine.

---

4 One of the most graphic examples of this was a clinic visit. My mom woke me an hour and a half before we were to drive down to the clinic to give me a Gravol to alleviate any symptoms I might feel on the drive down. Instead of feeling ready to go when we were supposed to leave, I was tremendously groggy (I needed assistance to walk anywhere, to get dressed, etc.) and felt extremely nauseated. This was at exactly the prescribed time for the Gravol to be working. The drive to the clinic was sickening. Mom and Marian sat in the front seat as I tried to sleep painfully in the back. An hour later, while still driving, the Gravol had worn off. I sat up and felt immeasurably better. In this case the anti-nausea pill had caused me a lot of discomfort. We stopped using it after this episode, relying on ondensetron and natural remedies instead.

Still, I was nervous about trying anything that might interfere with the chemotherapy and cause it to be ineffective or create unexpected and undesirable reactions. So I started thinking about introducing some non-allopathic interventions without any biochemical base, such as relaxation, meditation, and therapeutic touch. I had read Norman Cousins (1979) and knew his theories of laughter and vitamin C.[5] Herbert Benson (1979) wrote about research on the relaxation response. Larry Dossey (1993, 1996) had written about space, time, prayer, and healing. Deepak Chopra (1989) wrote on ayurvedic medicine and meditation. I had read some of the reports in the Western press on Chinese medicine and had followed, from a bit of a distance, the development of the theory and practice of therapeutic touch (Wager, 1996).

When we were still in the hospital I asked a friend to make relaxation tapes for Lauren. She asked Lauren where her favourite place in the world was and asked her to describe it. The tapes were then custom-made and used audio images from Lauren's cottage memories. They were beautiful but didn't work too well for Lauren: when she wasn't at the clinic or feeling sick from the treatments she wanted to escape in the way she knew best, by watching television and videos, and, of course, she was also doing homework for her five classes. Understandably, that was all the 'concentration' she wanted. Although we listened to these tapes a number of times, they never became useful to Lauren and we generally fell asleep sometime after the first few minutes.[6]

And so I turned to therapeutic touch. It is a non-invasive, non-chemical intervention the major obvious result of which is the elicitation of the relaxation response. This is a process in which the healer moves his or her hands over the body of the person who is being healed, at a distance of about 3–6 inches in smooth motions. The theory behind this treatment method is that the energy fields that surround living organisms can be 'smoothed out' and this will

---

5 Mom and I rented all the Steve Martin films we could find one week and had a blast. We did exactly what Cousins had described. It was fun and relaxing!
6 I feel that they were useful in this case. It helped me relax enough to sleep, which is also helpful, though not in the same way as meditation.

stimulate a healing process. Besides speeding the healing of wounds, there is also evidence that it can cause hemoglobin levels to rise and improve specific functioning in the immune system (Wager, 1996). In fact, one of the things I had wanted to do on this year of the fellowship was to learn therapeutic touch, and I had heard that there were two good teachers in town. Lauren and I both signed up to take the first course. She sat with her head on my lap, really too sick and tired to listen or practise. After two weeks, she had a fever and was admitted to the hospital. I missed one night but finished the first level and began practising right away. Whereas listening to a tape didn't work for Lauren, she was willing to sit still, often just to eat her breakfast while I gave her a therapeutic touch treatment. Before long she found that she took the opportunity to meditate, to visualize and affirm her well-being while I did therapeutic touch. Each treatment lasted just a few minutes, but I usually did it a number of times every day—in the local hospital, when Lauren was admitted for two weeks at the end of January for intravenous antibiotic treatment for a fever and neutropenia, I seemed to do it about six times a day, and later, at home, perhaps three or four times daily. The best thing about therapeutic touch for us was that Lauren was willing to sit still for it, for short periods, and did relax during it.[7] I, too, found it of benefit. I felt more relaxed both while I did the therapeutic touch and afterwards.

Lauren was diagnosed in mid-October. By mid-January I was giving her regular therapeutic touch treatments and looking around for other non-invasive help. From what I understood, there might be other 'natural' treatments that could be of benefit to her, that could help balance different parts of her whole system and minimize the side-effects of the treatment. The problem here, though, was to find a good, expertly trained, and experienced practitioner who had helped people in our situation, particularly young people with cancer. I just didn't know how to locate such a person. I looked and looked in the Yellow Pages. I read books and articles from the library.

---

[7] At first I just participated in these sessions with Mom to please her. However, after a wound on my arm healed much more quickly than I thought it would I started to believe in it more. I started to use this time productively, too, in prayer and meditation.

I called and talked and listened to various people about the alternative, complementary care they knew about or were giving. It was just so hard to know how to evaluate the options: how to choose. One mistake I made was to call a woman with a Ph.D. who had a relatively large advertisement in our local phone book. She apparently offered acupuncture, and because acupuncture was not a chemical intervention yet had good supportive research on its efficacy with certain bodily processes, such as pain reduction and, I hoped, nausea control, I was interested in pursuing it as a possibility for Lauren. So I called and asked about her training, her certification, her Ph.D., and what type of practice she had. She was very anxious to help and said that her son had been healed of lymphoma about 10 years prior with completely natural treatments and that she had people praying for all her patients. Her enthusiasm won me over and I made an appointment.

Full of hope, Lauren and I went to her office. Perhaps I should have known to turn around and walk out when I saw the huge book entitled something like *Who's Who in Ontario* opened to her name, the sort of 'vanity' publication for which one sometimes must pay to be included. But I thought I was jumping to unwarranted conclusions, so Lauren and I sat and waited while the receptionist said good-bye to a patient, sold him some pills, and, among other things, indicated that he wasn't to eat iceberg lettuce but only leaf lettuce. Still, we waited in hope for the doctor. Then, from an internal office, erupted the worst cough and throat and chest clearing I had ever heard. I had explained, as I was always explaining, that Lauren was intermittently neutropenic and was therefore vulnerable to infections. When I heard this coughing I got up and asked the receptionist if that was the doctor. When she answered yes, I indicated that Lauren and I would have to go because she was neutropenic. We left in a sleet storm and headed home.

Next I called an old friend/acquaintance who had just graduated in naturopathic medicine. I was ambivalent about this because I knew that part of her treatment repertoire was herbal remedies and I was still concerned about biochemical interference. Yet, I knew that she was interested in offering complementary care for people who had been diagnosed with cancer. So I called her, explaining that Lauren had leukemia and that we would like to talk to her about the ideas that she might have for adjuvant therapy. I said we were nervous about trying anything that Lauren would ingest but wanted to know what the possibilities were and what the research indicated. This was in March, and I was still afraid about drug interaction possibilities and afraid to mention to the doctors at the clinic that we were being 'unfaithful' and looking around for more help for Lauren—for the side-effects and for the strengthening of her whole system.

The naturopathic doctor met us with a typed two-page prescription of herbal alternatives and their purposes for specific organs (spleen/liver/pancreas and kidneys), for immune functioning, and for strengthening her blood. A number of her suggestions were easy to incorporate into Lauren's diet. Artichokes, for instance, were a favourite food. They were also useful. Rosemary as a tea or as a spice was suggested. Apricots were recommended. There were other things that were a little more obscure, but she suggested that Lauren could be helped by simply adding a few foods to her diet. We thought about it and decided to try some for three months to see if there were any benefits. We'll never know whether any of this helped or not, but we believed it might. And so, even if only as a placebo, these dietary supplements might have been of some benefit.

Complementary/alternative health care was not discussed as an option in the clinic. At no time did a doctor or a nurse take the initiative of asking whether or not we were trying non-allopathic adjuvant therapies. Each time complementary medicine had been mentioned it was in the context of a warning. We understood the message to be that using non-conventional treatment could be dangerous and so we had better report any deviance. We had been told that folic acid and some vitamin pills, especially some B-complex vitamins that are often included with folic acid, might alter the effectiveness of other prescribed drugs.

This approach to the use of non-conventional treatments is problematic. The effect is (likely) to discourage people from being honest. Not to make conversations about non-traditional methods a routine part of clinic visits is to ignore potentially valuable information for understanding the effectiveness of the prescribed allopathic protocols. Pediatric oncology is a field with increasingly successful prognoses. However, it is still not perfect. Everyone does not live. Besides, the side-, after-, and late-effects of the various drugs and the radiation can be severe and even fatal.[8] If the differences between those who 'do well' and those who do not are related in any way, either positively or negatively, to the use of adjuvant non-conventional care, it is important for all concerned to document its impact.

This assertion makes sense because we know that many people who are well, as well as people who are ill, use non-conventional medicine. In what has quickly become a widely cited study, based on a 1990 telephone survey of a national sample of the (healthy) US population 18 years and older, Eisenberg et al. (1993) found that one in three Americans had used at least one 'unconventional therapy' and that each American made an average of 19 visits to practitioners of non-allopathic medicine in the previous year. The researchers limited the therapies included in the study to the following sixteen: relaxation techniques, chiropractic, massage, imagery, spiritual healing, commercial weight loss programs, lifestyle diets (e.g., macrobiotics), herbal medicine, megavitamin therapy, self-help groups, energy healing, biofeedback, hypnosis, homeopathy, acupuncture, and folk remedies. The significance of these rates of seeking out alternative therapies is perhaps made clearer by the population estimates extrapolated from these findings. They indicated that there were more visits to unconventional than to allopathic health-care providers in the 12 months prior to the survey and that the amount spent 'out of pocket' on unconventional therapy was about equivalent to the amount spent for all hospitalization. This research, already almost a decade out of date, indicated widespread use of alternative medicine by a large percentage of the 'well' American population for health promotion and disease prevention.

---

8   These effects, not the disease itself, caused me the greatest anxiety. I know now what the side-effects are that occur with treatment. But what are the future ones? They are still a mystery. However, I am strong now and plan on continuing to exercise, eat well, and develop a meditation/prayer/journalling routine that works for me. I will work with my body to make it as strong as possible for the future. I don't believe that I will be sick again. But then, I never thought I would be in the first place either.

Studies of people with a variety of more or less serious diagnoses also reveal high rates of use of unconventional medicine. Yates et al. (1993), for example, found that 40 per cent of respondents in a sample of 152 people who had been diagnosed with a 'terminal' cancer and who had a life expectancy of two months to two years used complementary medicine. Other studies using varying methods of data collection and differing lists of treatments report complementary alternative therapies among cancer patients ranging from 16 per cent (Downer et al., 1994) to 54 per cent (Cassileth et al., 1984).

Several recent Canadian studies provide insight into the attitudes and views of allopathic doctors concerning unconventional treatments. One study (Verhoef and Sutherland, 1995), based on a questionnaire mailed to general practitioners in Alberta and Ontario, found that more that one-half felt that unconventional medicine could be of value for conventional medicine, with 56 per cent agreeing strongly that alternative medicine includes ideas and methods from which conventional medicine could benefit. When asked what alternatives they thought might be useful, 71 per cent said acupuncture, 59 per cent chiropractic, 55 per cent hypnosis, 34 per cent osteopathy, 17 per cent herbal medicine, 16 per cent faith healing, 12 per cent homeopathy, 9 per cent naturopathy, and 7 per cent reflexology. At the same time, most doctors said that they knew very little about any of these alternatives. Those they claimed to know most about were chiropractic, acupuncture, and hypnosis, where, respectively, 28 per cent, 24 per cent, and 23 per cent 'claimed to know a lot or a considerable amount about it'.

A similar study in Quebec (Goldszmidt et al., 1995) indicated that 59 per cent referred patients to physicians who offered non-traditional services and 68 per cent actually referred patients to non-traditional practitioners. These figures compare to different studies in Britain, in which 36 per cent, 76 per cent, and 59 per cent of doctors indicated that they referred their patients for non-conventional medicine (Reilly, 1983; Wharton and Lewith, 1986; Anderson and Anderson, 1987); New Zealand, where 80 per cent of physicians referred (Hadley, 1988); and Israel, where 42 per cent referred (Schachter et al., 1993).

A recent article in the *Canadian Medical Association Journal* stated that 'physicians must become familiar with complementary therapies, must inform their patients that they are available to discuss these methods, must be compassionate and non-judgmental and must direct patients to appropriate sources of care and information' (LaValley and Verhoef, 1995: 49). Eisenberg et al. (1993) drew a similar conclusion and noted that this generally did not happen: 'our observation that the majority of users of unconventional therapy did not discuss this therapy with their medical doctors suggests a deficiency in current patient-doctor relations.'

Why would I search for alternatives? Why had we always gone to alternative doctors and health-care providers? I understood that conventional medicine was a product of a particular time in history as well as a particular place. It is a modern and Western development, sometimes called allopathy because of its tendency to treat through opposites: i.e., surgery is to cut the problem out, chemotherapy is to eliminate the bacteria or other problematic condition, and other treatments such as radiation are basically designed to rid the body of the invader. Breast cancer activists have come to describe the current modalities of treatment for cancer as slash, poison, and burn.[9] The term 'allopathic' is used as a comparison to homeopathic, a system of medicine in which illness is treated with small doses of that which normally would cause the illness or problem (e.g., the antidote for poisonous snakebite is made from the venom of that kind of poisonous snake). In a homeopathic system the goal of treatment is to stimulate the body's own natural move towards health by simulating the symptoms of which the suffering person is complaining.

Western allopathic medicine has demonstrated enormous success with acute conditions. In the late 1930s and 1940s the promise of Western medicine seemed infinite. People who were mentally ill and who had formerly been incarcerated, bound into beds and

---

9 Although all procedures (I hope) are done as humanely as possible, the effect is severe. These treatments are all administered very hygienically and with rigorous standards ensured. However, these three words—slash, burn, and poison—feel accurate in their descriptive power.

chairs, and forced into strait-jackets were suddenly able to be 'managed'. The discovery of psychoactive drugs that worked to calm patients seemed to be almost miraculous at the time. Similarly heralded was the discovery of antibiotics, at about the same time, because these new 'wonder drugs' were able quickly to cure diseases, such as pneumonia, that had formerly been life-threatening. These successes, coupled with the growth in the legitimation and power of science and technology in the larger society and the association of medicine with science, gave medicine the patina of the modern and the advanced.

It has taken a number decades for the population to begin to see that allopathic medicine, by virtue of the particular models of the body and disease that it holds, has limitations. It is one way to look at, prevent, and cure disease, but it is not the only way nor is it necessarily always the best way for all sorts of conditions. Moreover, because of the sometimes severe side-effects and after-effects, it may at times cause more difficulties than it is able to cure. Indeed, it is well established that conditions that elude cure and become chronic tend not to be well managed by allopathic medicine because its focus has been on cure.

It is not just conventional medicine that has limitations; all schools of thought, rooted as they are in the particularities of history, economics, politics, technology, and the like, reflect a specific and limited focus. The problem with our ready acceptance of the positivist science and allopathic medicine is that it does not allow alternative visions. Its goal is to find universally true, objectively measurable causal laws. The point that I am making is a direct challenge to the epistemology of conventional medicine, and therefore may be read as a rejection of the whole of this tradition. However, that is not my perspective. Each school of thought, much as each disciplinary area of knowledge in the university where I teach, has a contribution to make to the growing knowledge that we have about any and all aspects of the world. At the same time, each provides only a partial understanding.

In my area of study, sociology, for example, there have been a number of useful pieces of research on mental illness. This research suggests that social class plays a role in causing and in treating mental illness. It also shows how the experiences of men and women within the medical care system result in different rates of different types of diagnosis of mental illness and, indeed, different types of treatment for these types of mental illness. Interesting and valuable as this sort of information is, both as knowledge in itself and with respect to social policy, it does not provide an understanding of why one individual rather than another suffers the symptoms of mental illness or is diagnosed and requires treatment for mental illness. The perspective of psychology is necessary for beginning to understand the causes and cures of mental illness on an individual level.

The point I am making, then, is that conventional medicine and its positivistic scientific basis has a very important role to play in providing an understanding of how our bodies work, and in diagnosing and providing treatment when they do not work—but other useful schools of thought and practice can add to this knowledge. Conventional medicine has a particular model of illness that can be called the 'medical model', which is 'based on the assumption that disease is an objectively measurable pathology of the physical body that results from the malfunctioning of parts of the body. All diseases are eventually explainable through a close analysis of the biological components of specific individual human beings' (Clarke, 1996: 302). In this model individuals are interchangeable with one another. This means that the treatment is for the disease and not for the individual with the disease. An upper respiratory infection is, for instance, treated in a basically similar way no matter whose upper respiratory system is involved. The old joke about the doctor referring to a patient in the hospital as the gall bladder in room 101 reflects this perspective. I should say, too, that I am making an oversimplification and overgeneralization to draw out points of comparison between this and other models.

Allopathic medicine claims to be based on positivist science. Positivist science is the science, developed in the last century and expanded in this century, that seeks universal truths through experimental research design. Its goals include objectivity, replicability, and generalizability. Positivist science claims to be above culture and social structure and unaffected by their vagaries. A great deal of research by social scientists with an interest in how knowledge, including scientific knowledge, is affected by social conditions shows how this claim of positivism is open to refutation. Suffice it to say that science is affected by culture in all manner of ways. For example, what gets taken up as a problem worthy of scientific investigation, the tools and concepts used in any particular investigation, the interaction of the scientists in the lab, and the state of the technology and equipment available are among the things that affect science and findings based on science.

There are other models of science and other models of disease, illness, and the body. These other models broaden the basis for understanding, prevention, early detection, and cure. They include the environmental, lifestyle, holistic, spiritual, chiropractic, homeopathic, and psychoneuroimmunologic models, as well as models based on traditional cultures, such as the Chinese and ayurvedic models. The environmental model focuses on the contribution of such things as poverty, unemployment, pollution, racism, global warming, acid rain, and similar conditions that are, in part, external to the individual human body but that may have more or less effect on the individual body through a variety of pathways. For example, the rates of cigarette smoking, now an indisputable but not sufficient cause of some lung cancer, are correlated with social class and gender. Poor men and poor younger women are more likely to engage in cigarette smoking than people of other social categories.

The lifestyle model emphasizes the importance of choices and constraints in lifestyle and includes such aspects of lifestyle as diet, exercise, sexual habits, stress management, and seat-belt use. Public health messages and the Canadian federal government tend to focus on topics such as these. The provincial governments, too, have adopted various aspects of this model. There is considerable evidence that diet makes a difference in health outcomes. In particular, research has indicated the importance of low-fat and high-fibre diets for the prevention of certain kinds of cancer and heart disease. Some case histories also provide tantalizing motivation for a more thorough investigation of the healing capabilities of a macrobiotic diet, even in cases of severe and life-threatening diseases such as cancer (Lerner, 1994).

A holistic model points to the advantages of looking at each individual as a unique combination of body, mind, and spirit. This model suggests that illness can result from disruptions in any of these three aspects of a person's life. It also suggests that a problem in one area will affect each of the other two. In this model the individual human being is indivisible. Cure, too, demands that attention be paid to all three components. Balance, harmony, and equilibrium are terms used to describe the appropriate interaction.

The spiritual model, which encompasses both major religious traditions and New Age philosophies, draws attention to the ways that illness can be seen as a result of a disjunction in the relationship between the embodied individual and the world of the eternal universal. Practices such as prayer and meditation are consistent with this view of illness and have been found to be associated with improvements in health. Studies of both prayer and meditation, done from a positivist perspective, demonstrate the effectiveness of these two behaviours in the increase in health and wellbeing (Dossey, 1993, 1996).

The spiritual model is related to the energy model of healing and illness, except that the focus in the energy model is on the empirical demonstration of energy fields associated with all individuals as well as all things in the physical world. These energy fields are thought to be universal and to tie all of us together. If we are all composed of fields of energy and if these energy fields surround each individual outward towards infinity, then all matter is related to all other matter and change in any one energy field reverberates across the universe. The belief that the flapping of the wings of a butterfly in India can cause a tree to fall in Canada is an expression of this perspective. Therapeutic touch, polarity therapy, and the use of crystals are among the associated healing methods.

Chiropractic as a profession is a rather recent development of an ancient healing tradition based on the spine. Chiropractic is based on the assumption that the relationship of the spine and the nervous system to all other organ systems is fundamental to good health. Manipulation of the spine itself can allow the body to correct itself in other ways and without the use of drugs or surgery. Chiropractic views the body as a unified whole but claims the primacy of manipulating the spine for the overall encouragement of a return to well-being.

Homeopathic is another holistic theory of health and illness. In this case, however, the method of cure is through the administration of infinitesimally small amounts of natural substances that, in themselves, cause the same symptoms as the problem that they are designed to cure. Homeopathy relies on complex information based on the knowledge developed after the observation of numerous individual cases over more than a century. As such, it is based on empirical science but not on positivism. Positivism's search is for universally true causal laws explaining and predicting health and illness that would be applicable across time and culture. Homeopathic's search is for specific remedies for specific symptoms, for particular and unique individuals.

Chinese and ayurvedic medicine (the traditional medicine of India) both begin with very different models of the human being and his/her place in the world. They emphasize the importance of harmony and balance for the person in the world and focus on strategies for living a good life, such as diet, exercise, meditation, spiritual awareness, and attunement. As such, they are holistic.

My basic point is that it is time that allopathic medical science and practice recognize that people often use complementary and alternative modalities, in spite of the fact that they are not included (with some few exceptions, such as chiropractic and massage, and then, only for a few treatments) in Canada's medicare system. It is also time that these complementary and alternative medicines are studied scientifically so that their efficacy or lack of efficacy in different situations is understood. This brief introduction to a variety of models of health and illness is meant to suggest the presence of other possibilities for viewing health and illness.

CHAPTER 9

HOW HAS CANCER CHANGED YOUR LIFE?

In this chapter I want to talk a bit about the social meaning of cancer and what some have come to call its stigma. It is difficult to find a personal experience that Lauren and I had that would illustrate her experience of stigma or, indeed, to know with certainty that any of her experiences resulted from stigma. When she first returned to school bald and chubby-cheeked after her diagnosis and the early, most aggressive stage of treatment, Lauren felt the teachers and some fellow students ignored her or didn't know what to say to her. On one occasion three of her high school peers (boys she didn't know personally) looked away when she tripped and fell in front of them and cut and bruised her knees very badly. And I could describe what seemed to me to be stares and whispers when Lauren and I went out together during that first winter when she did indeed look sick. But I do not know whether these felt reactions were just my or Lauren's interpretation of a reaction to the stigma of cancer—or something else. I do know that Lauren looked like the stereotypical 'child with cancer'. She bore the physical realities of the disease and the reaction of people around her reflected this.

A local cancer support centre often, during the time of Lauren's treatment, advertised a scholarship for students entering university whose lives had been touched by cancer. Lauren had considered applying but in the end she was ineligible because it was for students entering university and she was in her second year by then. But when the essay topic was announced—How has cancer changed your life?—we both felt uncomfortable. What could be wrong with this question as a theme for a scholarship application?

The best short answer I can come up with is Lauren's quip, 'Why don't people ever ask how having had a root canal has changed your life?' I think that it has something to do with the stigma attached to cancer or, as Susan Sontag would term it, the metaphors associated with cancer. She says, 'a surprisingly large number of people with cancer find themselves being shunned by relatives and friends and are the object of practices of decontamination by members of their household, as if cancer, like TB, were an infectious disease' (Sontag, 1979: 6).[1] But it is not just the stigma that leads to avoidance and practices of contamination or infection control. It is also, and perhaps more so, the stigma that results from the association of the disease with the person's character. Thus the person with cancer is seen as somehow morally flawed, inadequate, and in need of redemption or at least change. The person with the disease is viewed as somehow responsible for her or his diseased state. As Sontag states, 'there is mostly shame attached to a disease thought to stem from repression of emotion' (ibid., 16).

Cancer is viewed as a disease that reflects the whole moral worth of the person. It is a 'four-letter word' (Clarke, 1985: 25). One of the popular theories about cancer causation is that it results from psychological malfunctioning. Lawrence LeShan (1977) and Carl Simonton (1978) are psychologists whose work on this topic has become classic and has been taken up by some of the more contemporary popular cancer self-help writers, such as Bernie Siegal (1986). Typical of his views, and somewhat of a bedrock upon which a whole tradition has been built, is the following description of what LeShan presents as an exemplary case:

> The emotional pattern of Catherine's childhood was typical of my cancer patients. In almost all cases, damage had been done to the child's developing ability to relate early in life, usually during the first seven years. From their experience at this time,

---

[1] Although Sontag's writing is a little outdated in terms of 'decontamination practices', her main point still seems to apply to what happened to me. People equate the word 'cancer' with death and thus are afraid. During my illness many people disappeared from my life. I do not believe this was because they had forgotten about me but rather that they were afraid for themselves and afraid of me. Who was I now? Did I look sick? Had I lost my hair? Was I throwing up all the time? Obviously, I wasn't the same me—for how could anyone with cancer be the same? I am sorry for their fear and I understand it. Now I know that the most important thing to do is to get over it anyway and write a note or call ... always practising this is the trick.

these children, who many years later would become cancer victims, learned to feel that emotional relationships brought pain and desertion.... loneliness became the child's doom. In the usual manner of children, their loneliness was attributed to some fault in themselves, rather than accidental forces or the actions of others. Guilt and self-condemnation were the inevitable response. (LeShan, 1977: 50)

Such theories did not begin with LeShan. In ancient Greek medicine, cancer was considered to be the disease of melancholy people. Today, psychological explanations and concomitant treatments abound, and several studies of the mass print media confirm that these ideas have spread beyond the professional psychologists to become part of common-sense folklore. One recent study compared three diseases of major significance in North America today: AIDS, heart disease, and cancer (Clarke, 1992). This study showed that the mass media today reflect similar attitudes towards cancer and may both reinforce and even help to create such attitudes. Table 5 portrays the comparative imaging of cancer, heart disease, and AIDS in the mass print media.

The implication of the question of how cancer has changed your life is, after all, a moral question. Is your life better now? Did cancer teach you a lesson? Have you been aware of and obeyed cultural dictates that suggest that cancer can and even should be a moral turning-point, the occasion upon which you realize the mistakes in how you had chosen to live previously and are now willing to reject your old ways?

Some social psychologists have found that most of us tend to believe, in general, that people tend to get what they deserve. As discussed previously, this has been called the 'just-world hypothesis' (Stahley, 1988). As a result, when bad things happen to people, they themselves may be blamed and seen as responsible. Fate is fair and, therefore, if an individual is suffering he or she must have offended fate. They were careless, reckless, or overweight. They smoked. With cancer, according to Sontag, the explanations often seemed to be associated with repressed emotions. As she says, 'many people believe that cancer is a disease of insufficient passion, afflicting those who are sexually repressed, inhibited, unspontaneous, incapable of expressing anger' (Sontag, 1977: 82). These explanations serve to reinforce, to the presently well and accident-free, the belief that they have control over their lives. Such a belief

Table 5
Images of Cancer, Heart Disease, and AIDS

CANCER	HEART DISEASE	AIDS
Cancer is described as an evil, immoral predator.	Heart disease is described as a strong, active, painful attack.	Little is said about the nature of the disease other than it debilitates the immune system. Much is said about the moral worth of the victims of the disease.
Euphemisms such as the Big C are used rather than the word 'cancer'.	Heart disease, stroke, coronary/arterial occlusion, and all the various circulatory system diseases are usually called the Heart Attack.	
Cancer is viewed as an enemy. Military imagery and tactics are associated with it. The whole self, particularly the emotional attitude of the person and the disease, is subject to discussion. Because the disease spreads and because the spread is often unnoticed through symptoms or medical checks, the body itself becomes potentially suspect.	The heart attack is described as a mechanical failure, treatable with available new technology and preventable with diet and other lifestyle changes.	Acquired immune deficiency syndrome is called AIDS. The opportunistic diseases that attack the weakened immune system are often not mentioned.
	It occurs in a particular organ that is indeed interchangeable with other organs.	AIDS is viewed as an overpowering enemy, as epidemic and scourge. It is described as affecting the immune system and resulting from mostly immoral behaviour—connotes 'shameful sexual' acts and drug abuse.
Cancer is associated with hopelessness, fear, and death. Prevention through early medical testing is advised.	There is a degree of optimism about the preventability and treatability of the disease.	
	The heart attack is described as very preventable. Suggestions for lifestyles that will prevent it are frequently publicized.	It is associated with fear, panic, and hysteria because it is contagious through body fluids, primarily blood and semen.
There are innumerable potential causes listed. They range from sperm to foodstuffs to the sun. There is little consideration of the sociopolitical or environmental causes, e.g., legislation that limits smoking.	There is a specific and limited list of putative causes offered again and again. There is little mention of sociopolitical causes. There is certainty about cause.	Prevention through monogamous sexual behaviour or abstinence and avoidance of unsterilized needles and drug abuse.
		Initially the causes for AIDS were very general: being homosexual, a drug user, or a Haitian.
There is uncertainty about cause.		There is little mention of sociopolitical causes.
		There is uncertainty about cause.

Source: Clarke, 1992.

is comforting to hold—that we have control over our lives and can continue to prevent bad things from happening.

The derogation of the victim is well documented. Indeed, sufferers themselves may ask how they caused their own misfortune. This may serve to offer to the victim of misfortune some potential sense of control. Before the appearance of AIDS, cancer was the most feared disease in North America (Stahley, 1988). It is likely still the most feared disease among the largest segment of the population. This is because AIDS is still, although erroneously, thought of as a 'gay' disease and to a significant extent limited to homosexuals. Perhaps surprisingly, many medical personnel also believe the cultural stigmas associated with different illnesses (Stern and Arenson, 1989).

Stereotyping is not confined to adults with cancer. Several studies have demonstrated that even among the most educated of us, children who have been diagnosed with cancer are stigmatized. It is difficult to observe or measure the effects of a cancer stereotype in 'naturally' occurring interpersonal relationships between those with cancer and others. Such a participant-observation study would be expensive and time-consuming. Moreover, some of the reactions we would be observing would be due to the effects of the treatment on appearance, such as hair loss, weight gain or loss, and changes in facial features, including the chubby cheeks that sometimes result from ingestion of the steroid drugs frequently included in the standard treatment protocols. I certainly think that I observed the effects of cancer's stigma in Lauren's life when she had leukemia. I remember that it was routine for people to stare at Lauren when she had lost her hair, when her cheeks were swollen and she looked sick. Whenever we were in public I observed people scrutinizing Lauren. Perhaps some of the avoidance behaviours of some of her teachers and friends were related to stigma. Lauren remembers going to a restaurant after her graduation formal—to which she had worn a svelte black shift dress and a bald head covered in sparkles—and having people 'gape'.

One study of perceptions of children with cancer involved undergraduate and medical students who were asked to observe videotapes of four- and five-and-a-half-year-old children. The children were playing with an assortment of toys. Students were told that two of the children were in remission from cancer and two were healthy. Each child was, in fact, healthy. There were, nevertheless, clear differences in how the differently labelled children were perceived. 'Children described as in remission from leukemia, and free of the manifestations of the disease for several years, were perceived by both undergraduates and medical students as less sociable, less cognitively competent, less behaviourally active and less well behaved, less physically potent, less mature in their physical appearance, and less likely to adjust well to the future than the children described as healthy' (Stern and Arenson, 1989: 601). Since the only difference between the children was the label they were given, the label itself must have been the cause for the different perceptions. It is important to note, too, that the sample is composed of highly educated people and includes future doctors.

In a follow-up study the researchers developed and assessed an educational intervention designed to mitigate or eliminate negative stereotypes associated with childhood cancer among first- and fourth-year medical students (Stern, Ross, and Beilass, 1991). As a preliminary step the researchers compared the attitudes of the medical students in the first and fourth years to see whether the medical education served to ameliorate the negative stereotypes held in the first year. Initially, there was no difference between first- and fourth-year students in their attitude towards or biased beliefs about children with cancer. Even fourth-year students who had completed a rotation in pediatric oncology maintained cultural stereotypes. However, they did find that information-based intervention, which consisted of reading a description of the positive psychosocial sequelae of cancer, had the desired effect of minimizing stereotyped attitudes of those students who had read the material.

Ironically, perhaps, the stigma associated with cancer, in this case childhood cancer, seems to be perpetuated in the related research literature. This is noticeable in the assumptions behind what is taken to be important to investigate. If the medical, psychological, sociological, and epidemiological literature perpetuates myths and misconceptions, it is no wonder that medical students and doctors at times adopt these perspectives. This bias is found in the research literature on how people respond to a cancer diagnosis. For example, it is assumed that the parental search for understanding cause stems from guilt. As one group of researchers claimed, 'for parents, the search for cause and meaning is closely tied to feelings of guilt because parents have the practical and moral responsibility for the children's well-being; a child's suffering, illness or injury calls into question the parents' child-rearing capabilities' (Ruccione et al., 1994: 72). Further, 'parents *appropriately* respond with feelings of helplessness, fear, anger, guilt, and sadness' (ibid., emphasis mine). Of course, such responses are normal and appropriate when there is any threat to the parent's child.

Even the focus on adjustment to a childhood cancer diagnosis, it would seem, is inherently based on the acceptance of a stigma. If not because of the 'unique meaning of the disease', why would researchers examine this disease specifically? Severe illness, serious accident, or other significant health challenges in a child must all demand adjustment and adaptation for a child as well as the family. There must be many common issues for children and families, whether the diagnosis is cystic fibrosis, muscular dystrophy, paraplegia or quadriplegia resulting from a severe accident, or any of a number of other challenges to the body. Wouldn't it be more fruitful, for the development of theories about adjustment to diagnosis and ultimately to coping with chronic medical care, to consider the similarities and differences of all such 'challenges' together?

Another example, reflected in the research literature of the way in which cancer is thought to be a unique disease, is in the focus on the assumption that people react to news of a diagnosis with the existential or moral questioning of why me? In fact, there is a virtual research industry devoted to how people answer this question in the face of a serious diagnosis. By now, it is assumed to be the first response to catastrophic news. Some researchers try to predict its answer to later adjustment and coping (Taylor, 1983).

The notion that people make causal attributions when confronted by a sudden or unexpected calamity is an idea with substantial support in the social psychology literature concerning both adults and children (Kleinman, 1988; Taylor, 1983). In *They Never Want to Tell You: Children Talk about Cancer,* David

Bearison, a psychologist who interviewed children of a variety of ages about their experiences with cancer, reiterates this viewpoint. He comments: 'how children resolve this question of why me, therefore, is a projection of their struggle to attribute meaning to an emotionally painful and seemingly arbitrary series of circumstances' (Bearison, 1991: 123).

The question of why me, or why Lauren, was never a question I asked, at least not in a moral or existential sense.[2] I did not wonder what I had done that was morally wrong or what Lauren had done that was morally wrong. I did not think that it was either my or Lauren's essential being that had brought on the disease. I was curious about what there was to know about the causes of leukemia, about the incidence of childhood cancer, about the treatments, their side-effects, length, and frequency. It seemed clear to me then, as it does now, that the reason that anyone, at any time, succumbs to a serious illness or accident is always the product of a multitude of forces operating together, and a great many of these are beyond individual control.

However, as a medical sociologist and an outsider to the personal experience of life-threatening or life-changing illness or accident, I had taken the experts' opinion seriously. 'Why me?' always had seemed to me to be something that I could understand being asked by a person in such circumstances. The research literature that I had read made intuitive sense to me. I had no doubt that this was a significant component of the experience of (and the adjustment to) catastrophe. Now I think that this may be an outsider's perspective and projection. Perhaps the assumption that one of the most important issues faced by a 'victim' (and the sufferer of the catastrophic event or illness is often called just that) results from survivors' 'guilt' and need to justify to themselves—to explain why this terrible event has happened to someone else.

The answer to the 'why me?' question may best be understood

---

2 The question of 'why me?' was not raised in my mind until post-treatment. It is now that I am dealing with the loss of those two years. At the time I was surviving and that was all I had energy for. We were being positive about my illness. I felt guilty about being sad for I knew I would survive, which was more than could be said for some.

by a different sociopsychological concept—the just-world hypothesis (Lerner and Simmons, 1966). This view, as discussed earlier, explains that catastrophic illness is the psychosocial responsibility of the individual. In a sense, the sufferer is blamed for his or her misfortune. He or she has experienced loss, is unable to express anger appropriately, or denies feelings.[3] This repression of strong feelings that are assumed to be associated with grief or anger is taken to be the catalyst for cancer (LeShan, 1977). This is the frequently argued hypothesis that Susan Sontag critiques so creatively in *Illness as Metaphor*. Health promotion discourse, another dominant discourse, may be used to 'blame' the sufferer. It uses slightly different dimensions. In this case disease results from over-eating, over-drinking, smoking, lack of exercise, and other lifestyle choices.

My critique does not mean to deny that there may often be social-psychological and lifestyle correlates of disease.[4] Rather, the points I want to make are that, as true as each of these theories may turn out to be, they are each only a partial picture of cause. Today, when I read the literature on causal attributions made by patients and parents in work such as that by Bearison et al. (1993), I find it difficult. Now, as I see it, the assumption is that when people become patients (or parents of patients) they all become alike and perhaps somewhat less than they were and in need of 'understanding'. 'Understanding' in this case is appropriated through the process of making the thing (or person) to be understood as 'other'—something other than or different from the person who has the capacity to do 'understanding'. The patients and their loved ones also seem to be described as if they have lost their abilities to think and reason. Their own 'stock of knowledge' is dismissed or ignored. As the fol-

---

3 The feeling of guilt for a patient can be overwhelming. I have thought at times that if I had not been so involved, so intense about my school, then I would not have become ill. However, I counter this with the truth that four-year-olds are the most likely to have my diagnosis and it is absurd to think that their lifestyle (i.e., stress) contributed directly to their illness. Also, I knew others who had much more stressful existences who were not sick.

4 However, as Mom stated above, a chain-smoking, meat-eating, non-exerciser could live longer than a herbal tea drinking, vegan, health fanatic. There are so many variables to consider it is impossible definitely to prevent cancer.

lowing quotation illustrates, 'as threats from illness increase in severity, patients have an increasing need to fabricate beliefs about the reasons for their illness; furthermore, the irrationality of their beliefs increases in direct proportion to the seriousness of the illness' (Bearison et al., 1993: 48, from Bard and Dyk, 1956).

Certainly, one of the things I thought about and that Lauren and I discussed was the extent to which there were accepted causes of childhood leukemia. The conclusion I came to, as an educated but not medically or epidemiologically trained person, was that the cause was undetermined. As a thoughtful person who reads the newspapers and science magazines and who is generally at least somewhat aware of the world around us, I believed that, had there been a single or even a few clearly correlated factors for all childhood cancers (such as radioactive fallout), I would have already learned this. I also knew that even if there were a few clear correlates from epidemiological research, the proof of causality was complex and required stringent tests. In addition, if a few factors were indisputably linked to leukemia in children the ultimate model would have to include multiple explanations and, indeed, multiple levels of explanation. Moreover, I expected that the specific causes or correlates would necessarily vary somewhat from individual to individual.

My own 'causal attribution' was that it was a mystery that Lauren was diagnosed with ALL. Causes were just not known or understood yet. We asked the pediatric oncologist what he knew about the causes of ALL, and he said that 'they' were not sure. Without looking at the research, I expected, because of the line of questioning that Lauren underwent at intake, that genetic correlates were taken seriously. I also knew that while it was true that my mother's mother had had two young children die of cancer, there had been other children in that generation, more than 30 in the next, and approximately 10 in the next generation arising directly from this genetic line. No one else had been diagnosed with cancer in childhood. Clearly, a simple causal model of inheritance did not fit: genetic inheritance is not a sufficient cause of childhood leukemia. And so answering the 'why me?' question inevitably involves having all the information necessary about the environment, genetics, biochemistry, social psychology, and ultimate meanings. I did not have—nor does anyone have—all this information. The answer that came to mind most obviously, then, was—the cause remains a mystery.

I now find the notion that as a parent or patient I would necessarily make ignorant causal attributions out of fear and anxiety to be problematic. Bearison et al. (1993: 48) go on to say that 'in a culture such as ours, which emphasizes cause and effect relationships and justifies medical treatments based on causal explanations, our ignorance about the causes of childhood cancers is difficult for patients and parents to accept.' Here, I would agree. Innumerable studies have been done on factors ranging from viruses to pesticides to electromagnetic lines. The findings are contradictory and confusing. None meets the ultimate criterion of causality, which includes a combination of both necessary and sufficient reasons for the occurrence of an event. It is hard for me as a parent and citizen to accept that, in spite of so much research and, indeed, so many preliminary yet promising findings, we do not know more about the causes of the disease.

One group of researchers has suggested that the types of causal attributions made are related to the styles and the effectiveness of different styles of coping. While they do say that those who do not make causal attributions tend to cope more positively, they suggest that this is because of their 'acceptance of the physician's statement that the cause of cancer is unknown' (ibid., 50). I also now consider this to be a demeaning statement because it dismisses the knowledge of parents. At one time the gap in education between doctors and the majority of the population was great. However, most people in Canada now go to some post-secondary educational institution, many are studying or working in a scientific field, or at least reading science magazines and journals on a regular basis, and many others know more or less about the scientific method and the problems of establishing proof of cause. To assume that people respond naïvely with existential, moral, and personal causal attributions is a form of patronizing. Morbidity and mortality are the result of a complex interplay of a number of empirical factors, such as those related to the genetic predispositions of the individual and to social and economic position, physical environment, and lifestyle. Neither well-being nor illness could be understood by a simple recourse to the existential questioning behind the 'why me?' question.

Although I am now very critical of the socio-psychological literature on attribution, there was a time when I thought it both valuable and intriguing. Then, it seemed to me to reflect a deep compassion and intimacy with the thoughts and feelings of people who were suffering from an unexpected calamity. In fact, I recognized that I often questioned myself about why I was sick with the short-term influenzas or colds that I had sometimes had. I believe it likely that this compassion and empathy motivated such research. I can surely understand that people might sometimes look at Lauren through the eyes of cultural stereotypes and stigma. I can understand this both from the perspective of one who felt her daughter may have experienced it and also from the perspective of the stigmatizer. You may find it shocking or surprising, as I do, but when I watched Lauren in her aquatics class during the first months of treatment, saw her bald head and chubby cheeks and her thin body, I felt something akin to horror. Through the distance of a glass window, I saw Lauren not as herself but as a 'pitiable creature'. My own stigmatic reaction to Lauren must reflect a deeply embedded cultural belief.

Chapter 10

Treatment Ends?

On a number of occasions we received contradictory information from the different doctors and nurses. Sometimes this felt life-threatening. Two of the most worrisome times occurred at two 'ends' of treatment. The first was when Lauren's prophylaxis intensification phase of treatment (a term used for the most aggressive period of treatment after the remission induction) was coming to an end. We asked one doctor when it would be over. He indicated that it would happen once Lauren had received the maximum amount of adriamyecin as determined by the protocol. Because she had missed so many 'week one' treatments he calculated this to be probably, approximately, sometime in the late fall about one year after her remission induction was complete (based on her prior rate of receiving adriamyecin). Lauren's nurse also indicated that this second stage of her treatment would be over in the late fall, according to the same criteria. We were expecting this forecast. The next week at the clinic, however, the other doctor and his nurse were on duty. They each indicated that she would definitely be finished in August. We queried this, because we had been given different information previously. We were spoken to sharply, as if we were stupid for having received the wrong information. At this point our sense of anomie was about as high as it ever was. If they didn't know when Lauren was to end the particular stage of treatment, how on earth could we trust that they knew what they were doing in other ways?

I decided that we needed a second opinion. By this time I had learned the name of another highly respected pediatric oncologist in another city. (I had been calling around to various friends and contacts.) I wanted a second opinion from him. So I asked Lauren's dad to call the hospital where Lauren had been receiving her treatments and speak to a staff doctor about this. The doctor questioned why we would want a second opinion several times. Richard said that it was because we thought it was the responsibility of parents to be sure that their child was getting the best treatment possible and that, no, we didn't have any complaints. Richard explained that we knew treatment at the big city hospital was excellent and that we simply felt it was our duty to ask another expert. After several reiterations of this position he seemed mollified, agreed with Richard's position that a responsible parent would behave thusly, and acquiesced to our seeking the opinion of the doctor in another city.[1]

At this point I called this other doctor in another town and at another hospital. He called back to say that he was going on holidays—could the questions wait? I said yes, except for one question. I explained that what I was urgently concerned with was the amount of adriamyecin that Lauren was to receive. By November we had estimated that she would have received the entire amount required by the protocol—by August she would have received 78 per cent. This doctor indicated that, at his hospital, they never give more than 55 per cent of the total amount prescribed in Lauren's protocol because of possible side-effects and long-term consequences. At that, we were satisfied to let Lauren finish the stage-two treatment in August 1996 prior to receiving the final measure of adriamyecin described in the protocol. This was just one situation in which the opinions of the doctors conflicted and the patient and the family had to find a way to make sense of the contradictions.

Many times over the course of the treatment we talked about how long it was going to be and about what we would do when we were no longer tied down to the twice-a-week hospital visits—one day for blood work, the next for chemo—and to the recurrent anxiety. The feeling of vulnerability lessened over time, but the dependence on the twice-weekly hospital visits did not. One drug, the steroid, dexamethasone, continued to play havoc with Lauren's emotions over the whole course of the treatment. Initially, while in

---

1 The outcome of this interaction was most assuredly in part due to the fact that my father is male. Also, my dad has a very good manner in negotiating with other people. He was a champion debater in university and so knows the skills required to persuade.

the hospital for the remission induction stage of treatment, the massive doses of this drug gave her nightmares. She would wake in the morning only to feel that she had not rested and that her sleep had been populated with frightening demons and dragons. One of the most terrifying of the images that she shared with me was being in bed with corpses and unable to rest or find room to sleep. As time went on, she was switched to a milder dose of the drug but it continued to give her problems. She felt as if she was in a fog and was confused and unable to make decisions a lot of the time. She felt depressed and lacked her usual enthusiasm and hope. This turned out to be one of the most difficult parts of that cycle, if not the most difficult. For five days in every 21, Lauren felt the effects especially strongly. The rest of the time she felt them, too, but at a lower level of intensity.

Lauren looked forward to the end of the emotional cycle with a great deal of hope and in anticipation of living without having to make allowances for how she might be feeling on any given day or week. For example, while in her first university term Lauren tried to schedule assignments such as essays to be completed at a time when she was not receiving dexamethasone. We dubbed the experience being 'dexed' and talked of avoiding scheduling all sorts of things during this time, particularly tests and examinations.[2]

The end of treatment, as long as it was a distance in the future, was anticipated with great delight and hope. The idea that the treatment lasted a specified time and that then Lauren would be finished was, at times, a comforting sort of knowledge. As the time for the end of treatment came closer and closer, however, probably during the last three months or so during the fall term of 1997 at school, I began to get anxious. Ironically, we had come to depend

---

2   For me 'dex' (as we call it) was the major negative force in my treatment. What it meant was simply this: after about two days on dex I would start to become confused and depressed for a range of 7 to 12 days. My mind felt clouded over, smothered, like someone had come along and dampered the world around me. As it started to affect me, I could feel the gradual creeping sadness. As it left my body, I could feel it lift a little the first day, then more the next, and so on. Every two weeks the world seemed fresh and new. I was happy again. As my treatment progressed the amount of residual dex increased in my body, leaving me depressed for a longer and longer time. Dex served to rule many of my days throughout my illness.

on these awful drugs that were both making Lauren sick, in one way or another, and, we came to believe, keeping her alive. The end of treatment loomed ahead in these last months of the protocol as some sort of free fall. As time drew nigh I was increasingly concerned about the future.

In the last few weeks or so before Lauren was to end treatment according to what we had been told at the time of diagnosis, I began to call down to the teaching hospital to talk to the doctors about when they expected Lauren to be finished. There had already been a number of serious differences of opinion about Lauren's treatment and I wanted to start working on getting a good and consistent answer before the hypothetical conclusion of treatment had come and gone. It took three weeks to arrange to see a doctor at the clinic and by that time I had made upward of 10 phone calls. We had been asking at our local clinic all along and they had not heard anything of a date for the last treatment.

A day or two before we were finally to go down to the teaching hospital to discuss 'the end' with one of the doctors who was in charge of the protocol, we heard that someone (one of the nurses, we learned later) had called the local clinic to see where Lauren was in her treatments and whether she was finished or not. This was a little disconcerting because the caller was from the place where the treatment was supposedly being directed. In any case, we went to see the doctor. We at last caught up with him, after a half-hour delay, when we asked that he be paged. He walked into the room with a big smile on his face and said very warmly to Lauren, 'Congratulations, you are finished your treatment.'

This did not sit very well with me because I knew she was in 'week two' (and that someone had called to our local out-patient clinic from his clinic asking whether Lauren had finished her treatment yet, just a day or two earlier). I jumped in and said, 'Oh no, she has not, she is in "week two". How can she be finished if she had her "week two" drugs just two days ago? Surely, the plan would be that she would finish this cycle. Besides,' I said, 'I would like to understand how and why you have made a decision to finish treatment when Lauren has not had all of her drugs.' In one of the previous phone calls I had asked the doctor to calculate the dosages in order to make a good and rational decision about termination. I wondered how she could be finished if she hadn't had all of her drugs. We knew that she had missed a certain number of treatments all along and that some of her dosages had been cut down. He said that the pharmacist had calculated the dosages and that Lauren was finished. I said that by those criteria Lauren could not be finished, as I knew there were a number of missing drugs. So I said that the pharmacist could not be correct. He then said he would go and call.

He left the room, and when he returned he explained that it had been impossible for the pharmacist to get all of the information because Lauren was being treated elsewhere. I said that could not be true because I knew the local nurse had faxed the information to the supervising hospital every week, so they actually should have known the percentage of each of the drugs that she had taken. 'But,' I said, 'if you have not received them I will immediately drive home to our local clinic, pick them up, and drive them back again.' The doctor replied that he would get the numbers and I said that we would be down next week to discuss the results of his evaluation and calculations. I asked if he would call around and get the latest advice on whether to continue the drugs until she had finished the amounts initially prescribed, even if it meant another six months (or more).[3] I also asked if he would do a search of the research literature for the latest thinking and empirical results on this matter.

Obviously, I was very anxious that this decision be made on the basis of the best of the wisdom available at this time. My anxiety was justified, I think, by the fact that we had been told that since Lauren had missed so many drugs all along she was no longer able

---

3   Can you imagine how I was feeling? We arrived at the hospital, my mom, my dad, and I, expecting to hear that I would have at least another few weeks of drugs. However, my doctor first tells me I'm finished. After a momentary elation, I started to cry. How could this be right? My mom started to ask questions and I continued to cry. This was not the way it was supposed to be. For once, everything should have worked out all right. As soon as my mom started talking about six more months I could hardly bear it. My doctor had said I was done—couldn't we just leave it at that? ... However, I was scared that I hadn't gotten enough treatment and that my doctor didn't even know. Obviously, we needed more answers.

to be in the clinical trial of the protocol. A clinical trial, it should be noted, is a research study that uses patients and a specific treatment protocol to answer research questions such as: What are the most effective drugs for attaining a desired outcome? Is it better to give those drugs intensively over a shorter period of time or less intensively over a longer time (in terms, for instance, of side-effects)? If the treatment is changed too drastically it may not be relevant for answering the specific research questions. Since Lauren no longer fit into the treatment plan we had all agreed to two years earlier, it seemed to me we needed to have a logical and empirical basis for ending the treatment at the same time as if she were still included in the study.

After this confrontation I called a number of times before this doctor finally got back to me. And then, it would appear, he only returned my call under duress because I had called and called. He still did not have an answer. Finally, I turned to our local and by this time much admired pediatrician at the local clinic, asking if he would try to help. He had been reluctant to get involved earlier and had encouraged me to try on my own to get the information. But by then he knew that I had made many phone calls and he knew the results of these calls. He said, 'I'll get back to you on Wednesday [this conversation occurred on a Monday] and if I haven't, call and bug me.' Tuesday he called me. He had spoken with one of the supervising pediatric oncologists who by this time reported that he had spoken with several other researchers in the field. The consensus seemed to be that Lauren was to finish on schedule regardless of how much of the drug protocol she had missed. Our local pediatrician was satisfied with this information and knew and respected the experts who had been consulted. He said that we should leave it as suggested. We did.

At the end of treatment, much anticipated though it was, we felt an anti-climax. This was true not only because of the shifting sands regarding the decision as to when the treatment would end, but also because it was not over yet—we visited the hospital less frequently, though not for treatment but for check-ups.

By the time the treatment ended Lauren and I were so comfortable with our twice-weekly visits to the local clinic that we missed them and the cheerful conversation with people who knew what Lauren was going through and who were regular cheerleaders for her progress. Saying good-bye to this routine, which after almost two years had become a lifeline, had both positive and negative aspects. On the one hand, it was wonderful to be at the end of the weekly assault of the cell-destroying and mood-altering drugs. On the other, we were leaving behind what had become a comfortable routine of visits, jokes, and warm embraces—and birthday and other seasonal celebrations.

This decision that treatment was over occurred after Lauren had finished, but we didn't know it at the time. The last treatment passed as just one more treatment because we had not heard yet from the supervising doctors regarding when to stop. We have half-wondered a number of times whether or not Lauren would still be on treatment if I had not called down to the supervising cancer centre to ask when it would be over. The question seemed to throw people there into motion—but once again, a motion of contradiction and confusion.

In one of the conversations with a supervising doctor around this time I had learned that only 1–2 per cent of all children in this protocol receive all their drugs. A second piece of new and valuable information was that the point of treatment is to keep the counts low. This I took to mean that if Lauren's counts were too low to receive treatment on some scheduled weeks, that was all right because it meant that the leukemia cells were not growing either. I am not at all sure, however, about whether that is what was meant. If it is true it would have been of incredible help to know this earlier, as it would have relieved a great deal of anxiety. Getting information from the doctor was so difficult that I did not have the heart to try to pursue the question so that I could understand the ramifications of the comment that the point of treatment was to keep the blood counts low.

The end of treatment is psychologically very important to parents and children. As Keene (1997: 355) says, 'many parents describe ending treatment as almost as wrenching an experience as diagnosis. Families begin to experience the gamut of emotions—from elation to terror—months before the final day.' Further, she notes that 'generally on the last day of treatment a child in remission from leukemia has a diagnostic spinal tap, a bone marrow aspiration, a complete blood count and chemistry screen, a thorough physical exam, and a discussion with the oncologist' (ibid., 357). Clearly, Lauren's 'last' day of treatment missed the mark.

We were not alone, I am sure, in the ambiguity that we experienced at the end of the treatment protocol. Not only is the time of treatment a traumatic, ambivalent time for the child and parents, but it is likely also the case for the doctors and nurses. They have often, I expect, gotten to care about and developed relationships with their patients. Coming to the end of a relationship for all of us always involves some sense of loss. The fact that the end of this relationship is also a source of long-awaited joy may make it more difficult to express the loss.[4] The unexpressed loss may make this time more problematic for medical staff than it needs to be. I know that at the end of every term of teaching at the university I feel a sense of loss. It doesn't matter whether the classes have been good or not. In fact, in a way my ambivalence about the end of the course is even greater if the class has been difficult in some way, perhaps because at the end there is no chance to make amends or finally to transform the difficulties. Just as a number of other components of Lauren's treatment for leukemia, the end to treatment was problematic.

After treatment ends patients are followed up for five years. For the first years, this involves biweekly visits to the local clinic for blood count assessment, along with monthly visits with the physician. Several times a year the assessments are more detailed investigations of such things as liver and heart functioning. For the second and third years after the end of treatment, blood count assessments occur monthly. Subsequently, for the 'final' two years medical assessment occurs four times per year. The follow-up schedule varies somewhat from protocol to protocol, but all children are followed for a number of years post-treatment. Seven years post-diag-

---

4   The pediatric nurses at the local clinic who treated me week in and week out will never know how much of difference they made in my life. The head nurse in the clinic, in particular, still makes me feel special and wonderful when I see her. These nurses knew that my life had much more to do with everything not related to cancer than with being a cancer patient.

nosis Lauren will be considered cured, which in the uncertain language of cancer treatment means that her likelihood of a cancer diagnosis would be no greater than that of another person her age, sex, and so forth who lacks her medical history.

What is it like to live with this ongoing uncertainty? Do we worry all the time, or every time a blood test is taken? Are anniversaries of the day of diagnosis still difficult? I don't think about the disease very much. Life has returned to 'normal', which is surprising even to me—the fear has abated. I seldom think of the past, and the intense feelings of the time quickly recede to dim memory. It is amazing how resilient people can be—or is it denial, as some psychologists might say? But anniversaries, such as diagnosis day, hair loss day, and the (approximate) end of treatement do remind me.

There is a whole other research industry on the psychosocial adaptation of survivors of childhood cancer and their families. The fact that this research exists confirms both the existence of some problems for some people and the assumption that problems are likely to continue. This literature makes the point that long-term adjustment for people with visible and functional effects (such as limb amputation and learning challenges) differs from that for those with no long-term effects. People who have had brain tumours removed and who have suffered some concomitant brain damage obviously experience long-term effects and changes as the result of the diagnosis and treatment. At the same time, those without functional effects, and their families, by and large do well on a number of different measures. This is especially significant because of the sizeable proportion of the population who are survivors of childhood cancer. As detailed in Chapter 3, it is estimated that by the year 2000, one in 900 young adults will be a survivor of childhood cancer.

Chapter 11

Cancer Charities for Kids: Answers to Dreams and Wishes?

Lauren eventually was able to inject herself with neupogen, the drug designed to stimulate the growth of white blood cells, which would hopefully enable her to receive treatment more regularly and fight off infections. Initially, however, a home-care nurse came by daily, at a prescribed time, to administer the shot. One of the home-care nurses, who was particularly kind, told Lauren about an organization to which the nurse belonged that ran a summer camp, Camp Quality, for children with cancer. She offered to give Lauren information about the camp and suggested that Lauren might like to attend. This nurse subsequently dropped a camp brochure off at our house. Lauren contemplated going to the camp, but before the time for deciding on whether or not to go arrived, another 'opportunity' presented itself through this same organization. This was to be a day-long trip to Disney World for 'kids' with cancer and their siblings, as well as the siblings of children who had died of cancer. Each 'kid' with cancer was to have a companion for the day. Ever ready to try something new and to take part in whatever was happening, Lauren decided a one-day trip to Florida was not likely something that she would experience again, at least not in the near future.

There were medical forms to fill out, summer clothes to find, hat and sunscreen to purchase. Eventually the day arrived when Lauren was to go to a hotel in Toronto, stay overnight, and leave at about five o'clock in the morning for the airport and the three-hour flight to Florida. Lauren was still in the early consolidation days of her treatment (this was in May, about seven months after her diagnosis), and she felt quite sick and tired when she awoke at the hotel in the morning. She was ambivalent about going to Disney World in this condition and wondered if she would be able to have a good time. All around her were younger children, both with cancer and not, but there did not seem to be anyone else in the early stage of active treatment. (It is in the early stage—the first year or so—that children can be easily indentified by their lack of hair.) The one young woman there who was her age had finished treatment a number of years earlier and was, by this time, quite healthy. The only other people who were her age were companions of others, and they all seemed to be in the bloom of very good health and pleased to be able to help out a child with cancer and, besides, get a flight to Disney World for a day. The healthy companions were doing what many well teenagers would be doing on a day and night away from their homes—they were having fun, partying, flirting, and making lots of noise.[1] Lauren did not really belong here. She was neither well enough to party with the 'companions' who were her age, nor young enough to have fun fooling around and playing with the pre-teens and younger children.

Being too sick and too old, however, was only a part of the difficulty, as it turned out. Even though she didn't feel well Lauren decided to go to Florida, despite the fact that the home-care nurse who had first told her about the camp, and had observed that morning that Lauren was not well, offered to stay with her at the hotel, to swim and relax for the day. As a true adventurer, Lauren decided to go and the home-care nurse decided to go with her and be her companion for the day.[2] Off they went to the airport at five in the morning to be met by cameras, reporters, and bags of gifts and treats including candies, toys, and games, many stamped with corporate logos. Much to Lauren's chagrin, it appeared that the reason they had to rise so early was to be interviewed and photographed so that the donor's generosity would be recognized and widely

---

1 I slept in a room with three other girls and women who were all well known to one another and who had not seen each other in a long time. Thus, the talking did not cease until two in the morning. I had been used to being in bed by nine and sleeping until at least eleven the next morning, so three hours of sleep did not quite cut it.

2 I was miserable that morning. Early mornings were very hard for me throughout the full course of my treatment. I felt nauseated and out of sorts. I wasn't sure if I was going to be able to make it. However, I felt that by not going I would somehow have failed, because I didn't know that I was the only one who was still on active treatment. I thought that there were others in my situation and that I needed to 'get over' my morning illness like everyone else had.

known. Lauren said that she spent the day being pushed around to different sites while sitting in a wheelchair. Because some of the chemotherapy drugs and the radiation made her particularly sensitive to sun at this time, she spent a lot of time under the various trees that dotted the landscape, covered with sun-resistant clothes and a big sun hat. She felt really tired and unwell all day and realized at the end that she probably shouldn't have been there. In fact, the home-care nurse who had recommended Camp Quality and this trip told me later that she cried when she returned home and told her family how badly she felt for having taken Lauren when she was feeling so poorly.

It turns out that this experience is just one of many similar examples of 'the ways and means' of the children's cancer 'charities' industry. We had already experienced a few manifestations of this huge, behind-the-scenes effort during Lauren's earlier days of hospitalization and treatment.

Within the first week or two, while still in hospital, we were told about the Ronald McDonald House. This is a hotel-type service that provides space for families with a child who is being treated for a serious or life-threatening illness. There is a nominal fee for use of facilities, which include rooms for all sorts of activities such as sleeping, eating, playing, being entertained with television or music, talking and visiting with other families.[3] In an early conversation with one of the nurses on the ward, and emphasized again in the clinic, the pleasures of Camp Trillium were extolled. Shortly after we arrived home a quilt arrived from Project Smile. This organization was started in 1993 by a couple whose son had been diagnosed with ALL when he was two and a half years old. Their little boy, Matthew, while he was undergoing treatment, had carried everywhere the quilt that his mom had made especially for him. As a result of this experience Matthew's parents decided to develop a project that would provide quilts to children diagnosed with cancer in Ontario. I had not spent much time thinking about childhood

---

3 My dad and Marian stayed at the Ronald McDonald House and quite liked the atmosphere and privacy it provided. However, since they were only staying there for a short time and lived so close, the service was not really a necessary one for them.

cancer before Lauren was diagnosed. I remember feeling 'touched' by the kindness of the anonymous people who had made the quilt for Lauren. It seemed such a generous and caring gesture, made as it was by strangers, that for a few moments, and even now when I think of it, the world seemed a better place.[4] There was also an organization from which we received a newsletter almost as soon as we returned from the hospital—'Candlelighters'. This turned out to be a recently established outgrowth of the Canadian Cancer Society. Its mandate was the establishment of and support for parents' groups across the country, as well as a national association to operate as an umbrella organization for parents' concerns and to hold biannual conferences. Candlelighters also supported Inter-link nurses, who would provide specialty care for children being treated for cancer at home, school re-entry programs, and many other initiatives. These are just a few of the charities of which we were informed in the early stage of Lauren's treatment.

After the trip to Disney World, though, I began to question the world of cancer charities. I wondered how many charities were 'out there' for Ontario children. I wondered about the range of the kind of things they offered. Did they work together? Did they compete with one another? How did they choose their recipients? How did they get names of people with childhood cancers? How could we find out what sorts of services were available? I also started to wonder whether or not they were all legitimate. Once my eyes were opened to the presence of organizations such as the Children's Wish Foundation, I started to see and hear about a variety of children's cancer charities. I also began to feel uncomfortable about what started to look like a densely populated field of specialty organizations, most with 'heroic' goals associated with sunshine, rainbows, and wishes of 'special' children. It seemed large, confusing and complex. I began to wonder whose interests were being served by these organizations, and whose interests were being ignored.

---

4 This quilt is on my bed at home. It is beautiful. I was pleasantly shocked when I received it and still appreciate the donors' goodwill.

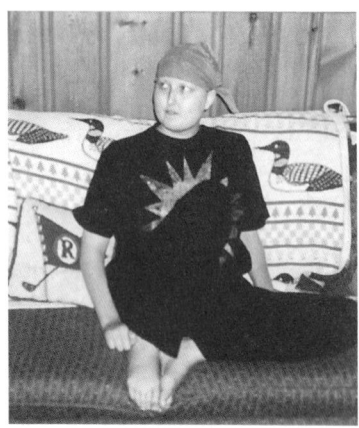
Lauren in a scarf that she sometimes wore in the early stages of treatment.

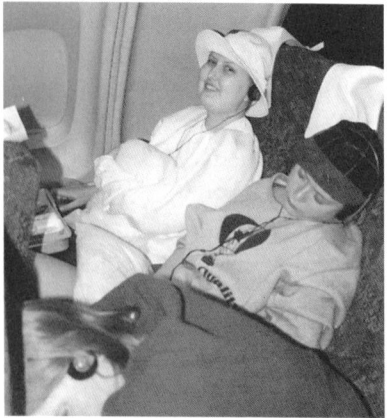
Lauren on the airplane for the Dreamlift to Florida and Disney World, May 1996.

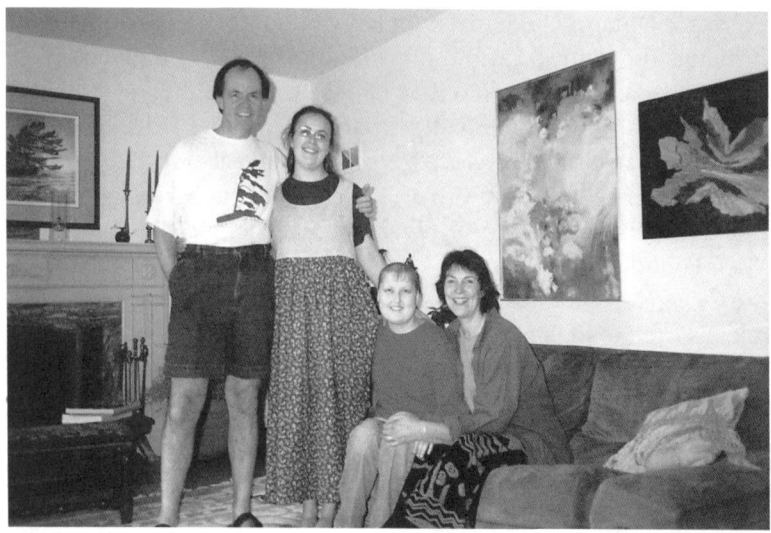
Richard, Jess, Lauren, and Marian at home, 1996.

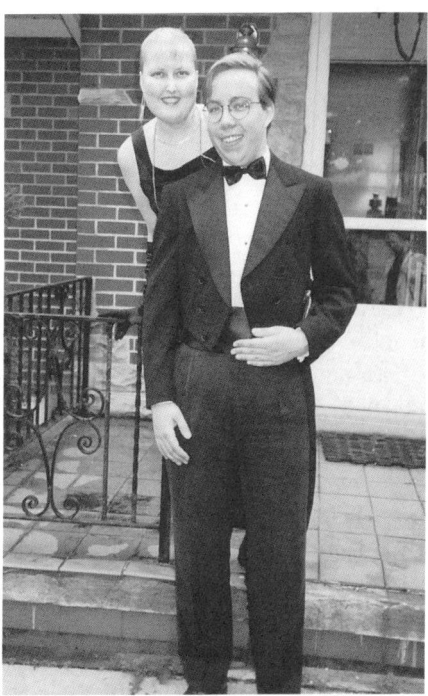

Lauren and Michael on their way to the prom.

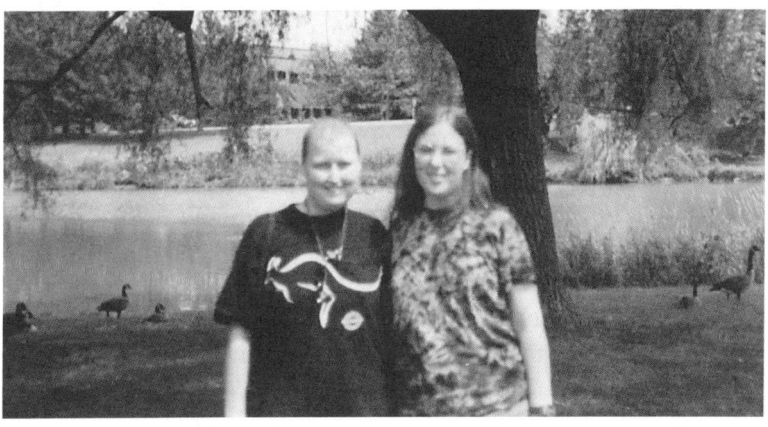

Lauren and Jess at Conrad Grebel College, just before Lauren began university and Jess went to Africa, summer 1996.

I decided to search for answers. Phone calls were made to the most well-known organizations. Each was asked to send information about their organization and if they knew of other organizations. We also asked how they make their services known both to the potential funding sources and to potential recipients of their funds. At the same time we asked if they could tell us what was unique about their organization. Using this process we discovered three different camps in Ontario: Camp Ooochigeas, Camp Trillium, and Camp Quality. In addition, there seemed to be a number of different 'wish' organizations through which children with cancer could have a wish fulfilled. These organizations had names like The Children's Wish Foundation, Starlight Children's Foundation, The Jennifer Ashleigh Foundation, Make-A-Wish Foundation, The Sunshine Foundation, Aladdin Children's Charity, A Child's Voice, Guelph Wish Fund for Children, and The Golden Griddle Children's Charity. These are the wish organizations discussed in this chapter. (See the Appendix to this book for further information and ways of contacting these and other organizations.)

This is, however large as it is, not an inclusive list. At the end of this painstaking process, in which we asked everyone at these organizations for the names of other organizations, I just happened to find a brochure of another organization at a local plaza and then saw a huge sign announcing fund-raising efforts for a different group again, associated with university students during frosh week at a local university. The list I have may represent most or just the tip of the iceberg. I don't believe there are any methods that would allow us to be sure that we have identified all of the organizations. This is in itself a problem. If it is very difficult for a person who is making a concerted effort to find the names and addresses of all of the organizations, how much more difficult must it be for parents whose children have cancer to connect with the right organization for help, advice, or to ease their burden, or, for that matter, for people who are administering such organizations or being asked to give money to know that the money will be spent in an accountable, responsible fashion without a needless duplication of goals.

The first step, after receiving brochures, application forms, and newsletters from these organizations, was to see what sorts of unique services they offered. It soon became apparent that there was a lot of money being raised and spent and that a number of the organizations had overlapping and potentially competitive mandates. These organizations do not appear to be shoestring operations. The Make-A-Wish Foundation, for instance, which claims to be the largest non-profit wish-granting organization in the world, proposes to fulfil one wish for a child under 18 who is suffering from a life-threatening illness. In southwestern Ontario alone the organization reported that it had raised over $600,000 and granted wishes to 130 children since 1985. (This is a small fraction of the number of children with cancer and other life-threatening diseases. From 1985 to 1992, for example, there were 3,511 diagnoses of cancer in children in Ontario [Hutchcroft et al., 1996: 87].) If all of this $600,000 raised in southwestern Ontario had gone to these 130 children that would have meant upward of $4,600 for each child's wish. Some of the wishes filled, according to a recent brochure, include, for a little boy with leukemia who wanted to be a police officer, a custom-made uniform, helmet, badge, and a ride in a helicopter. Another little boy with leukemia and his family were given a visit to Disney World and a chance to meet Mickey and Minnie Mouse. A 14-year-old girl with bone cancer wished for, and received, along with her mother and best friend, a trip aboard a cruise ship for fans and stars of the soap opera *Days of Our Lives*. I do not question that such wishes might have been a 'blast', as one recipient described hers, but we do need to ask whether this is the best use of the money available.

The answer to this question is complex and variable. It reflects one's basic values regarding distributive justice. Some could argue that this money is raised for these purposes because people want to give specifically to provide a little help or joy to an individual suffering child with a serious, life-threatening, or terminal disease. In this perspective, such donors would be less likely to provide money for research or for services such as art therapy, which might be given to a hospital or clinic for the use of a number of children. The same rationale, of course, motivates the fund-raising programs of various 'adopt-a-child' charities whose focus is health, education, and community development for the poor in developing or war-torn countries. By personalizing the appeal for money and appealing to the emotions of potential donors, fund-raisers with noble goals and good intentions have found they can have greater success.

To answer questions about fiscal responsibility, we asked for the annual reports, including financial statements and auditors' reports, from all of the organizations on our list. All but the Aladdin Children's Charity, whose spokesperson said it did not have such a thing, and the Golden Griddle Children's Charity, which refused to send its financial reports, did send the information requested. The Jennifer Ashleigh Foundation had only a financial statement, but it did send this along. All were asked for and all gave their charitable tax receipt numbers. The amounts raised varied tremendously, but the services did not.

As I investigated the question of financial accountability, I discovered that it was very difficult to compare one organization to another or to assess fiscal responsibility. I consulted several accountants, who indicated that disclosure and fiscal accountability to the public are not clearly mandated in either the public or private sector. In fact, some universities are just now struggling under public pressure to make their accounts transparent. However, I remained sceptical about the value of the childhood cancer charities industry for serving children with cancer. How can competing organizations maintain a focus on those they are designed to serve at the same time as they are competing with other organizations attempting to provide the same or similar services?

This is particularly problematic in the context of the disparate needs of children with cancer. Indeed, cancer affects children of all socio-economic levels but seems to affect poorer children even more harshly because they are more likely to die (Nelson, 1992). All children and their families suffer some economic hardship as a result of this diagnosis.

A recent study has documented the out-of-pocket costs to parents of children while they were being treated for three different childhood cancers: acute lymphoblastic leukemia, Wilms tumour (stages 2–5), and neuroblastoma (stages 3 and 4) (Barr et al., 1996). The researchers asked parents to estimate costs using both prospective and retrospective surveys. They distinguished among the three diseases because of the length of treatment, as well as the high, medium, and low survival prospects for each disease. The average total expenses (in 1986 Canadian dollars) for the duration of treatment for each disease was $26,070 for leukemia, $20,074 for Wilms tumour, and $10,376 for neuroblastoma. The researchers concluded that 'overall, in spite of universal first-dollar coverage for medical care in Canada, family-borne costs during the course of these illnesses are at least one-third of the average family's after-tax income' (ibid., 933). According to these researchers the costs included all of the following:

- food purchases while travelling to and from treatment sessions or during treatment sessions;
- special foods required for the patient;
- transportation required for patient care;
- accommodation near the treatment centre—even Ronald McDonald charges families a token amount (it was $10 per night in the community in which Lauren was being treated);
- long-distance telephone calls associated with treatment;
- drugs and medical supplies;
- professional consultations for treatment purposes;
- gifts, entertainment, or outings undertaken due to the patient's treatment or disease;
- clothing needed because of weight loss or gain by the patient;
- special equipment, including mattresses, wigs, walkers, wheelchairs;
- special purchases for patient comfort such as air-conditioners, humidifiers, vaporizers;
- additional vehicle or alteration of a vehicle to suit patient needs;
- vacations taken because of patient's disease;
- household modification because of patient's disease.[5]

---

5   We did not make many of these expenditures because I was mobile, because my weight loss was not overwhelming, because I did not wear a wig. However, I still know, with the special drugs I took, the days off of work that my dad took, the telephone calls, and the transportation to the medical centre, that we spent a lot of money.

Not only, however, does the family have extra expenses, but often one parent either has to 'quit' work or has to cut back substantially on hours of work. These wish foundations operate in the midst of the lack of such fundamental needs as palliative care in the home for the dying child, other home-care services, certain drugs, medical devices, and even medical procedures that are not covered by medicare (for example, I understand that the 'flushing' of the port-a-cath, a procedure done every three weeks to prevent infection and blood-clotting, among other things, at a cost of about $100 per flush, was recently privatized in Alberta). Families whose children have cancer must then pick up the cost or their children run the associated health risks. I continued to question the cost-effectiveness and value of such foundations to families and to their children with cancer. Are these wishes trivial—or are they important? Are these really children's wishes? Do they serve the best interests of children and families or not? This is a value judgement that I cannot make for everyone, but all should know the whole situation of inequality and unmet needs before deciding.

One person I spoke with, for instance, while quite critical of wish organizations in many ways, felt that at times they offered an invaluable service to the dying child and family. She was a bereaved parent whose family received a week-long trip to Disney World when their child was near the end of his life. She remarked to me that not only was it wonderful for the family to plan for and anticipate, but it has provided the siblings and parents with many priceless memories. A number of years later, they still remember that fun time just before their brother/son died. Cherished as this time and memory continue to be, even this mother was critical of what she thought was the frequent misuse of funds from wish foundations that could be better spent for many, many needed services for *all children with cancer*, such as art or music therapists at clinics.

Perhaps most important is the fact that the wish foundations in a sense compete with one another in marketing and fund-raising. To illustrate: Candlelighters is attempting to be the organization for the additional needs of those who suffer the effects of childhood cancer.

Candlelighters is now poised through extensive marketing, public education and fundraising endeavors to position itself in Canada as the organization which addresses the issues and needs of children and families living with the unique impact of childhood cancer and its treatment. (Executive Summary of Business Plan, 1997: 11)

According to its 1997 annual report (p. 2), Candlelighters' success has been remarkable: 'This past year has been one of unprecedented growth for The Childhood Cancer Foundation—Candlelighters Canada. We have witnessed the rapid expansion of our donor base which in nine months has increased from just over 1,000 to just under 60,000 Canadians who have made a commitment to children with cancer and their families.'

Many might argue in favour of this drive for a monopoly position being made by Candlelighters because its goals are national, and this organization is attempting to be need-based rather than wish-based. Nevertheless, it is clear from Candlelighters' documentation that the world of cancer charities is a competitive one.

I have asked the question, whose interests are served by these organizations? One answer is suggested by the dedication found in *Wishbone*, the newsletter of the Make-A-Wish Foundation.

To Our Wish Children
They touch our lives for just a little while,
They face tough odds with courage and a smile
We fly them to 'the stars' if that's their dream,
They teach us what joy and magic really mean,
We try to ease their pain and show we care,
They leave us treasured memories to share.

This is an example of the sort of appeal that these organizations make. To me, such imagery perpetuates one of the sources of suffering for those with childhood cancer: the stigma. This statement stimulates certain emotional reactions and reflects some of the emotions that are put to work (Hochschild, 1983), and perhaps exploited, by many who raise funds for childhood cancer. This is especially the case for those whose mandate is individual children and their wishes. Emotions are not natural, spontaneous, and free-flowing; rather, they are used in the service of culture and social structure. They are 'constructed' for use in many areas of everyday life. Some retail stores today have a greeter whose job is to make the shopper feel welcome. They are trained to and it is their job to do so. They are to use their emotions to express warmth, friendliness, and welcome in order to generate a feeling of well-being and enhance purchasing behaviour in the customer. By contrast, the expression of emotions such as sadness and grief is encouraged by the whispers, dark suits and cars, boxes of tissues employed by those who meet with families to arrange funerals and in funeral homes at the time of visitation. We all learn how we are to feel in various situations through processes of socialization (e.g., in school we are to style emotional expression in favour of rational or creative learning) and interaction with others (e.g., we learn not to laugh when a friend describes a sad experience). Charities, too, tend to be associated with, and hope to generate in potential donors, certain emotions—namely compassion, sympathy, perhaps even pity.

In the brochures of children's cancer charities, emotions are generated by the extreme pathos implied by the visual and verbal portrayal of smiling, courageous children who are dying young. Emotions are also created to 'help' these 'pathetic' children by giving them whatever they wish, even that most extraordinary gift—'flying them to the stars' to 'show we care'. In return, they are said to 'teach us what joy and magic really mean'.

We examined the brochures that were sent to us from the variety of wish organizations for language that seemed to be used to generate emotional sentiment. Some organizations, such as Candlelighters, were matter-of-fact and informative about their services and their needs. Most, however, used language to generate emotion and sentiment. Table 6 illustrates our findings.

One of the organizations describes its own 'Dreamlift' as a flight from a Canadian community for up to 80 'special children' to a dream destination such as Disney World for one day. I am not sure if this is the organization that sponsored Lauren's trip, but if it is I guess Lauren had a chance to make her 'dream come true' — although, in what appeared to be a full list, three 'Dreamlifts' that took place in 1996 were mentioned, but none was from Toronto in May. Possibly there is another 'Dreamlift' program. However, Lauren had been to Disney World several times, each time at a more leisurely pace and each time when she was well. I am not sure how appropriate it is to consider this particular one-day trip to Florida

Table 6
The Emotional Appeals of 'Wish' Organizations

Organization	Examples of Emotionally Appealing Language
A Child's Voice	• born out of a need to bring some joy • brave young victim • we salute and celebrate our beautiful 'children with cancer'
Starlight Foundation	• memorable wish—the little boy who wished for food for his family for a year
Sunshine Foundation	• I saw a little boy who couldn't speak. He had the most amazing look on his face. His eyes were filled with so much excitement that he seemed to be shaking with joy. I will never forget that look. For all the challenges he faced, none of them seemed to matter.
Project Smile	• make their lives brighter
Children's Wish Foundation of Canada	• for those children who may never have a tomorrow, there's the Children's Wish Foundation of Canada • Eric just cannot do what other kids take for granted; to run and play, Eric sits and relives his wish day after day.
Guelph Wish	• to relieve some of the pain, sadness, and turmoil caused by that illness
Make-A-Wish	• We strive to make each wish a magical experience so nothing is left to chance.
Golden Griddle Children's Charity	• golden sunny skies are just around the corner • an outstanding day that left everyone feeling good inside by realizing that they had made a difference in so many young lives • Matthew whose leukemia is now in remission was able to keep his grades thanks to his friends at Golden Griddle Children Charity.

her dream.[6] Yet, 'volunteers offer thousands of hours of their valuable time' in raising money for the foundation. The Canadian Forces, the Navy League of Canada, the Royal Canadian Legion, and various policing organizations such as the RCMP, the Ontario Provincial Police, and the Canadian Association of Chiefs of Police are 'official' partners. A variety of foundations, such as the Eaton's Foundation and the Sears Foundation (BC), are supporters. In 1996 the organization had more than $1 million in operating funds and over $600,000 in endowment funds. That is a lot of money. Is it well spent? Does it serve the interests of 'special children' or not? Are there negative effects of the effort?

Ronald McDonald's Children's Charities has provided capital funding for 12 Ronald McDonald houses associated with hospitals in Canada. In addition, they have contributed to the establishment of 197 houses in 15 other countries around the world. Each house is slightly different. Some provide housing and other services for oncology patients and families only. Others provide these services for families whose children have any illness that requires the parents to stay overnight, away from home, for a period of time. All of the operating expenses are managed by invisible volunteers, paid staff, and other individual and corporate donors. McDonald's Restaurants garner a lot of publicity and public relations 'points' for their houses, yet McDonald's contributes only seed money. The remainder of the money and the ongoing maintenance and services depend on the financial support of concerned community groups, corporate donors, foundations, and the general public. They also depend on the ongoing work of many volunteers. There are 130 volunteers in Toronto at the two Ronald McDonald houses alone. The contributions of these others is substantial in dollar terms. The 1996-7 annual report indicates that funds came from a 'variety of sources, including Special Events, the sale of Nevada tickets, Direct mailings, Memorial donations, Foundations and

---

6 It most certainly was not my dream. So, perhaps I should not have gone. In hindsight, I am not sure what we were thinking. I guess we thought that the nurse knew my condition and still thought it was possible for me to go. I also think I was searching for some relief (and even reward) for the suffering I experienced. This trip seemed to fulfil these desires. However, I was in no condition to travel.

Employee Group Grants, Tournaments, Capital Campaign pledge programs and fund raisers in the community held on our behalf' (Annual Report, Toronto's Ronald McDonald House, 1996-7).

CANCER CAMPS

The three cancer camps were each somewhat different. I will not discuss Camp Oochigeas because it is affiliated with and integrated into the care of children at one particular Ontario hospital, Toronto's Hospital for Sick Children. Camp Trillium is a member of an international organization of camps for children with cancer, Children's Oncology Camps of America. Established in 1984 in Ontario, Camp Trillium is affiliated with other oncology camps across the country, such as Kids' Camps of Alberta, and is governed by a board of directors that includes pediatric oncologists, nurses, social workers, and parents. It is also affiliated with the Ontario Division of the Canadian Cancer Society and the Ontario Camping Association. The camp is free to participants because it is funded by a variety of individuals, service clubs, businesses, and foundations, as well as by the Cancer Society. At least one experienced oncology nurse is on staff at all times. Safe transportation, including an emergency airlift to a nearby air base, and contact with the patients' oncologists are guaranteed. The camp is located close to a treatment centre and thus children can maintain their schedules of chemotherapy and radiation through visits from camp to receive treatment locally. Besides the medical backup, all of the counsellors are well trained and receive certification in CPR, first aid, emergency procedures, and water safety. The camper-to-staff ratio is 3:1, and different types and ages of camps continue all summer.

All of these medical facilities are in place in order that the children have fun and develop skills that all children learn at camp, including sailing, wind-surfing, canoeing, kayaking, swimming, fishing, camping, hiking, arts and crafts, and other such activities.

Camp Quality is a different type of camp. It is offered for one week only each summer. Campers may be patients, on or off treatment, or family members. Each camper is paired one-to-one with a buddy with whom the camper is intended to have a relationship over the year, from summer to summer. The brochure for Camp

Quality emphasizes that the camp allows 'children to be children again, to have fun, to make new friends, to participate in exciting activities and, as far as possible, to be removed from all stress'. Rather than emphasize the normalizing effects of a camping experience, as Camp Trillium does, Camp Quality emphasizes the extraordinary aspects:

> As a result, Camp Quality has touched the lives of many—campers, their families, volunteers and sponsors alike—over the past eight years. It is particularly rewarding to see the changes that the camping experience has made in campers' lives, and to see some of the campers return to be companions themselves.

The glossy 80-page brochure, filled with photos of campers and companions as well as camp activities, is titled 'Camp Quality: A Story of Hope'. It emphasizes that its major sponsor is Imperial Oil. Camp Quality in Ontario is one of 35 such camps around the world. It was established first in Australia, where there are now 13 camps in operation. What is not said in the brochure is that Camp Quality was established and continues amid controversy about its true purpose, its cost-effectiveness, and its safety.

In trying to understand this world of children's camps I made a number of phone calls and read numerous newspaper articles, only to find that Camp Quality is perceived as competition by many who support the oncology camps integrated with oncology centres. When Camp Quality first came to Ontario, I learned its local founders had had a number of conflicts with the camps already in existence. When asked to co-operate with the already existing camps, Camp Quality was reported to have said that 'they wanted to be the ones to help the children.' Rather than co-operate with the already established Camp Trillium in Ontario, the organizers set themselves apart, with their programming, their fund-raising, and their philosophy. The camp itself emphasizes that its funds come from 'a variety of sources, including individuals, corporations, service clubs and estates'. There is no mention of a church affiliation. In 1995 Camp Quality apparently had 46 campers for a one-week camp. The reported budget for the year was $60,000. Is this cost-effective?

One other concern about Camp Quality is safety. When children are in treatment they need to be within a short distance of a treatment centre. Treatment, in case of a 'bleed', for instance, should begin in a matter of approximately 20 minutes. With a fever it is advisable that a child who is neutropenic receive medical attention, often intravenous antibiotics, within an hour. Clear and open communication between the child's doctor, other pediatric oncologists, and the camp is also important. Camp Quality is neither close enough to a pediatric oncology centre to provide the desirable services nor linked closely and effectively with pediatric oncologists.

So far this chapter has raised, rather than answered, questions about the world of children's cancer charities. There is competition among them; the public relations may at times supersede the service to the children; there may be vested corporate or religious interests at work behind the scenes; there may be a lack of adequate protection for the health and safety of the children at times. Finally, an unintended consequence of the children's cancer charity industry may be the maintenance of the stigma of cancer. It is important, however, to see the children's cancer charities in the broader context of the charities industry in Canada, and thus as a way that Canadians have allowed social, health, and religious services to be provided.

Children's cancer charities, as unnumbered as I found them to be, are just a drop in the bucket of the charity sector across Canada. It is estimated that in the mid-1990s there were approximately 73,000 organizations registered with charitable tax status in Canada (Stewart, 1996) . Involving about $86 billion per year, or about 12-13 per cent of the gross domestic product, 'charity' is a bigger business than agriculture or the auto industry and employs more people than all three levels of government combined.

It is apparently very easy to become a registered charity. All that is required is that a two-page form containing a number of questions, most relating to names and addresses, be submitted. To qualify for charitable tax status the purpose of the organization must be charitable, which is defined as encompassing any one of the following four categories:

- the relief of poverty, including sickness and distress
- the advancement of religion
- the advancement of education
- purposes beneficial to the community. (Ibid., 6)

Once registered as a charity, a group can issue charitable tax receipts and begin collecting money.

Accountability is minimal. A charity is expected to devote its resources to charitable activities. Eighty percent of the income for which the charity issues a charitable receipt is expected to go to the charity—only 20 per cent is expected to go to administration and fund-raising (although the definitions of these categories are ambiguous). Charities are forbidden to advocate to change laws. Although each charity is expected to file a report documenting that 80 per cent of its income was spent on charity, Revenue Canada has the personnel to audit only about 600 charities per year. In the highly unlikely case that a charity is audited and found to be in violation of the law, the punishment is simply a revoking of the charitable status. According to Stewart, in 1994 about one in five—or 17,000 charities—did not file returns on time with Revenue Canada. Even those that did file on time frequently gave inaccurate or incomplete information. Of the 17,000 late filers, only three had their charity numbers revoked with cause; 237 withdrew their charitable status privileges. Further, those charities that did file returns claimed to spend, on average, about two-thirds of their income on charitable activities and one-third on administration and management—a clear violation of the 80 per cent/20 per cent rule (ibid., 7). Another investigation of the accounting of 20 health charities revealed an annual collection of $98 million, with $29 million spent on salaries and administration, $21 million on fund-raising, just under $49 million on charitable activity, and more than $35 million retained by the charities at the end of the year. These figures include retained income from the previous year (Corelli, 1997: 70). Supervising the ongoing operation of charities is the job of the provinces. Ontario is said to be the most effective province in this regard (Stewart, 1996). Yet there are only seven people in the Office of the Public Trustee to monitor more than 26,000 Ontario charities.

Cancer Charities for Kids: Answers to Dreams and Wishes?

There is approximately one charity for every 397 Canadians. Donations are both in money and in kind (e.g., clothing) and they are gotten through door-to-door canvassing, mail request, event sponsorship, place of worship, shopping centre canvassing, in memoriam contributions, payments to attend charitable events, and payroll deductions, among others. When asked, Canadians report that they give to charities out of compassion; to help a cause in which they personally believe; because they are personally affected by the cause that the organization supports; because they feel they owe something to the community; to fulfil obligations and belief; and/or for tax credit (Hall et al., 1998).

Of Canadians over 15 years of age, 88 per cent gave to a charity or non-profit organization between 1 November 1996 and 31 October 1997 (ibid., 13). Of these, 78 per cent were direct financial donations; 36 per cent gave change at a store check-out counter; 3 per cent left bequests; 63 per cent gave household goods/clothing; and 52 per cent gave food (ibid.). Charity bingos and casinos, a growing part of the economy, already total $409 million annually. Charity-sponsored raffles on lottery tickets comprise $463 million (ibid., 14).

There are a number of problems with this situation. The first is that as governments downsize the charity sector responds. There has been an increase of 5,000 charities over the past three years (Corelli, 1997: 68). The growth of the charity sector is one response to the privatization of health and social services. To the extent that the needed services are identified and efficiently and effectively delivered, whether or not this happens as the result of an obligatory tax structure or out of the goodness of peoples' hearts matters little. The problem arises because there is no way to track or evaluate the effectiveness or efficiency of such service delivery. In a situation that, to a large extent, lacks regulation and accountability, this is virtually impossible. Moreover, when services are mandated by a democratically elected government because they are believed to further the interest of the common good, recipients of service are entitled to these services—they are not, for all of the negative social meanings attached, 'charity cases'. And this can be the unfortunate, stigmatizing result when services become downsized, privatized, and ultimately charity-driven.

The field of children's cancer charities is probably made up of thousands of compassionate, kindly, and well-meaning people who volunteer time and provide money and goods because they care about and want, in some way, to minimize the suffering of children faced with serious and life-threatening illnesses. In the absence of regulation and accountability, however, competition among service providers, overlapping mandates, emotional manipulation of potential donors, waste of money, and even, in some cases, the provision of unsafe services are to be expected. When basic needs for all are met by government, then charities (in the children's cancer sector) can offer the icing on the cake. As long as basic needs are not met—and of course they aren't if mice are scurrying around the floor of a pediatric oncology ward—then the reliance on charities needs to be examined and recommendations need to be made. This is exactly what a recent group, the Panel on Accountability and Governance in the Voluntary Sector, established by the voluntary sector itself in 1997, has sought to do through a series of fact-finding, data-gathering procedures that include extensive discussions with relevant people and organizations. The panel's report, released on 8 February 1999, is under consideration by government at the present time.

CHAPTER 12

LOOKING BACK AND LOOKING FORWARD

This book has mostly been about a period of one year in our lives. It focuses on the time of the most aggressive stage of treatment for leukemia. The day after diagnosis Lauren's treatment—the initial remission reduction—began. Within a day or so the once lively young woman was sleeping most of the time, and when she woke up she felt exhausted and nauseated. As I recall, she vomited only about once a day. Those first weeks in the hospital were (and remain) a blur of days and nights folded together, of hope and anguish, of too many questions and too few answers, as were many of the episodes to follow. The accompanying chronology of events and symptoms (Table 7) helps to sort out all that happened during this time and later.

Table 7
Chronology of Events and Symptoms

Date	Significant Events/Treatment	Symptoms
Summer 1995	Lauren struggles to fulfil duties as counsellor at French day camp.	Fatigue, unable to hike, sitting in shower.
10 October/a.m.	To urgent-care clinic in town.	Continued tiredness, dizziness, palour.
10 October/p.m.	To hospital in big city.	
12 October	Diagnosis day.	
13 October	Remission induction treatment begins: in hospital for 30 days.	Virtually bed-ridden, exhausted.
31 October	Hair Loss Day.	
13 November	We move in with my brother Richard (L's Uncle 'Oily') in big city for 2 weeks, while radiation treatment is done and for intra-thecal chemo; 3-week cycles of CNS prophylaxis and intensification begin.	Exhausted, tired, nauseated.

Date	Significant Events/ Treatment	Symptoms
28 November	Radiation finished, we return home.	
January 1996	30 weeks of leg needle (L'asparaginese) begins.	Losing weight.
late January	In local hospital for 2 weeks to receive intravenous antibiotic.	Fever, neutropenia.
early February	Lauren returns to school for one class per day. The other courses she completes at home.	Losing muscle tone, palour, and quite weak, sometimes Lauren needed help to walk. At times she used a wheelchair to get in and out of the hospital.
22 March	Lauren's 18th birthday.	
May	One-day trip to Disney World.	Fatigue and nausea.
June	Leg needles (L'asparaginese) end.	Big relief to end one stage of treatment. Almost immediately Lauren began to gain weight and muscle tone and to feel better.
July	Confusion about when the adriamyecin would be finished.	
August	End of adriamyecin. End of CNS prophylaxis and intensification and beginning of maintenance therapy. And the end of the triweekly (or so) visits to the big city hospital.	Finishing adriamyecin was another big relief, started feeling a bit better.
September	Jess to Africa for one year. Lauren started first-year university at Conrad Grebel College, University of Waterloo. She took 3 rather than 5 courses. Still going twice a week to the local hospital.	For the next year and approximately three months Lauren experienced recurrent depression. Eventually this seemed to be about one week every three.
22 March 1997	Lauren's 19th birthday.	Lauren swam and did aquatics several times a week at her university pool.
May	Lauren began part-time work cooking in the cafeteria at Conrad Grebel.	

Date	Significant Events/ Treatment	Symptoms
July	Lauren experienced a severe sunburn on her feet after sitting in the sun (under the porch roof) for just about one hour.	Lauren's feet really hurt. She couldn't wear shoes and had to stay off work for almost three weeks.
September	Lauren started second year with 4 rather than 5 courses. She moved out of the house to live with 2 other young women in a townhouse adjacent to her college. We visited the local hospital twice a week and the big city hospital every three months or so.	Lauren continued to feel tired and to need a nap. But her hair was growing in, her muscle tone was back. She continued to exercise in an aquatics class and now walked to school and various classes.
November	The end of treatment. (We didn't know it was the end until afterward, so it was a bit anti-climactic.)	
22 March 1998	Lauren's 20th birthday.	
April	Port-a-cath was removed.	
September	Third year of university. Lauren's living with 5 other young women about a mile from school and she walks to and from her classes.	
November 1998	Lauren's Celebration.	She is 'back to normal' and feels well, although she finds she needs a nap most days (if she can find the time).

As the months passed during the first eight months or so of treatment Lauren's head remained bald, she was pale, with dark circles under her hollow eyes, and she lost more and more weight and muscle tone. She seemed to be disappearing before my eyes—her energy, her vitality, her strength, her enthusiasm, even her very body. Clearly, this process couldn't go on for ever. The drugs, it seemed to me, were killing her.

We looked forward to milestones along the way. One was the end of the weekly leg needle, the L-'asparaginese. Almost immediately, the end of this drug seemed to make a big difference. Lauren began gaining a bit of weight and muscle tone. Two months later, at the end of August and almost a year after the beginning of treatment, the adriamyecin was stopped, and again she seemed to improve remarkably. This drug was always associated with nausea and vomiting. It was the one that required the 'miracle drug' ondonsetron to keep the nausea and vomiting at bay before and during the whole period of the 48-hour infusions. It also kept her head mostly bald.

There were health scares during treatment. One time Lauren visited the dentist and had X-rays taken. When the dentist looked at her X-rays, knowing that she was under treatment for leukemia, he reported that he saw what must be a tumour beneath one of the teeth. He said that it needed to be investigated and he wished he had old X-rays. For a number of reasons, we had changed dentists not long after Lauren's diagnosis, but because we had recently changed this new dentist did not have prior X-rays. I asked if I could go and get these immediately. The dental receptionist called over to the former dentist's office and requested previous X-rays. I drove over and brought them back. I was terrified and so was Lauren. By the time I returned, the dentist had done some research with a text he had in his office and discovered that because of the shape and location, the 'tumour' was likely a 'calcification'. An examination of the previous X-rays showed the same 'calcification'. This confirmed his diagnosis and we were tremendously relieved.

While in the hospital during the remission induction Lauren had a terrible infection in the area of her wisdom teeth. A dentist visited and said that she would need her wisdom teeth out as soon as possible. Lauren was put on an antibiotic that was specific to this problem (along with all the other drugs). I was very worried about the prospect of Lauren having her wisdom teeth removed during the time of treatment because I was already anxious about her overall physical vulnerability, even without additional threats to her well-being such as those involved in the surgical removal of her wisdom teeth. Fortunately, she was able to finish treatment entirely before she had any recurrence of infection in the area of her wisdom teeth and that worry became unnecessary.

The first eight months or so after the end of the remission reduction—the prophylaxis and consolidation stage—was to be done on an out-patient basis. And it was, except for the two weeks in late January when Lauren had a fever and had to enter the local hospital for two weeks to receive an intravenous antibiotic. She was admitted locally a couple of other times, for just a few days with a fever. At least once, Lauren's counts were so low that she received blood over a lengthy period of time as an out-patient. This second stage of treatment was very hard. Lauren felt sick and tired virtually all day. She slept long hours. She couldn't go out with her friends because she was neutropenic or feeling sick so often. She seemed to be getting sicker and sicker, for days on end. I couldn't imagine her better. Then, with the ending of particular treatments, I began to see that there was hope and to believe she would get well.

Once off the L'asparaginese and adriamyecin, Lauren began the period of treatment called maintenance. During this time her hair grew—first to a fuzz, then a thin short crop. We laugh now because we thought her hair was back. Pictures tell a different story, as does her current thick head of medium long dark hair. The period of maintenance still involved weekly chemotherapy, but the drugs were far less toxic and so Lauren felt much better. Still tired and periodically depressed, she carried on through her first year at university, living at home and taking a reduced load of four rather than five courses.

It was difficult emotionally. She felt outside of the mainstream. She missed the excitement of moving away from home, of starting university, of being 'in it together' with others her age. She tried hard to be part of the school. Conrad Grebel, the college she attended, is a Mennonite college in the University of Waterloo. She took part in the weekly chapel service followed by a community supper, in which the faculty and all the residence students attended. But she was a triple outsider. She had not been raised as a Mennonite; she was not able to stay in residence because she needed sleep and treatment and could not be in such close contact with others as a result of her heightened vulnerability to viruses and bacteria that populate college residences; and she was sick with a life-threatening disease that required aggressive and sickening treatment.

We tried to find others in similar circumstances to talk with. I called the counselling office, the health office, the chaplain's office, and the local cancer support centre. None knew of others Lauren's

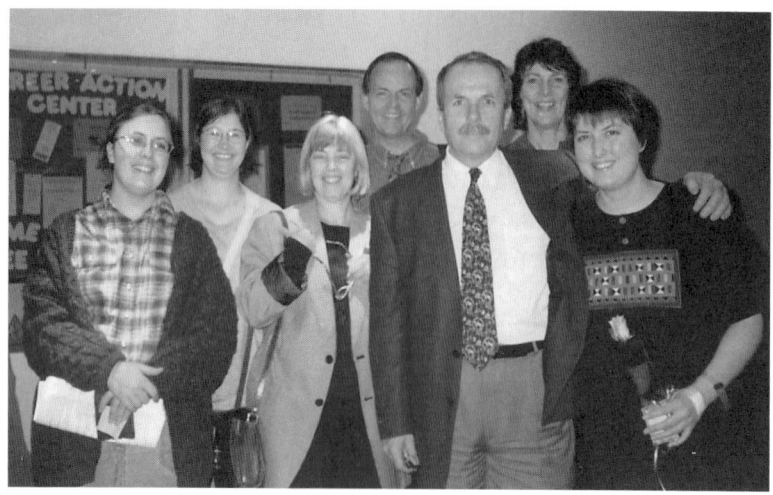

Celebrating the removal of the port: Jess, Beth (a friend), Juanne, Richard, Uncle Richard, Marian, Lauren, spring 1998.

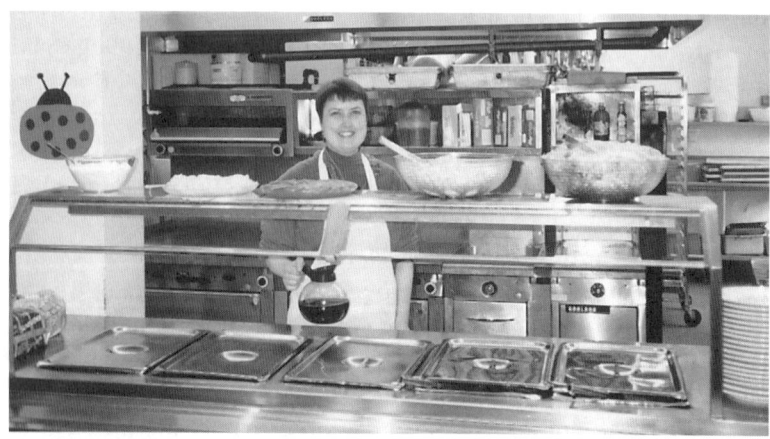

Lauren working in the kitchen at Conrad Grebel College.

age who were undergoing treatments. I called Toronto-Wellspring—another cancer support centre. This time we met with success. They had a group for 18–30-year-olds diagnosed with cancer. It was held every Tuesday night for a period of eight weeks, led by a psychologist and a 20-something 'survivor'. This group became Lauren's emotional lifeline. She started attending in January of 1997, when she was in her first year of university and on maintenance therapy. Tuesday nights became fun. We drove down to Toronto and had dinner together at one of the many downtown restaurants. I'll never forget her comment after she left the meeting on the first evening: 'I wish I could see and talk to those people every day.' She had been thirsting for someone her own age, people who 'really understood' because they were going through or had gone through a similar experience, with whom to talk.

I had been heartbroken as I watched her flounder emotionally, and lack her usual joie de vivre as she faced the future of university as an outsider to a myriad of common, taken-for-granted experiences of that first time away from home. I lived with sorrow day in and day out as I sat helplessly by. I drove Lauren to and from school, sometimes twice a day. I took her to the hospital twice a week and waited with her. I took her out to lunch, rented videos, took her to concerts. But I knew that there was so much more that she could and should be experiencing with her own friends.

We also experienced many particular new joys during this whole time of treatment. We developed close relationships with the nurses and the doctors at the local clinic. They were always and consistently supportive of Lauren. More than anyone else (other than family) in Lauren's life, they knew what she was going through. Both the pediatrician, who headed the clinic, and the head nurse had worked with children (and their families) with cancer for over a decade. They had seen many changes in treatment and more and more successful outcomes. And they were not oblivious to the dangers. We always felt exceedingly comfortable with them because they seemed to be very careful. We could see and hear them double-check Lauren's counts and the data sent by the big city hospital about her protocol and the quantity of drugs that Lauren was to receive at any time. If they were unsure about quantities they double-checked with the big city hospital. Lauren and I usually saw the nurses twice a week, and for most of the stretch of about 20 months she saw the same doctor about once per week. They knew about her interests in school, and in extracurricular activities; they knew about Michael and the prom (in fact, they posted on the bulletin board outside the clinic a picture of them taken before the prom with Lauren's almost bald head covered in sparkles). They knew about her sore and burned feet. They knew what she hoped to study in university, about her sisters' work in international development in Malawi. Lauren always felt cared for and respected. And I always felt that my worries and concerns were acknowledged and I was given relevant and helpful information and support. Not long after we started going to the clinic we began to celebrate birthdays—theirs and Lauren's—with special cakes and treats from a local bakery. So sometimes our visits seemed more like mini-parties than treatment for childhood cancer. I could hardly have imagined this but it is true—both Lauren and I have commented that we miss these visits. How can I thank or even say enough about the impact of this continuous support and excellent medical care? I can't.

Other joys included the remarkable generosity of so many people who offered flowers, cards, food, phone calls, offers of whatever help we needed, even for the long haul of the treatment period. One group of friends, when they heard that Lauren was sick, got together and organized a healing liturgy to which all brought candles and lit them for us. Later they brought the candles over and we had them burn for months after as a reminder of their love and concern. A number of my colleagues at work became closer friends as they lent a hand, or an ear, a practical service of a chance to escape to a lunch out, or something else to ease my preoccupation. Our church brought meals and flowers. Several people whom I didn't know well before this time always made it a point to say that they were 'thinking of' us regularly. One friend called a contemplative order of Carmelite nuns, told them the story of Lauren's sickness, and asked if they would pray for her.

Our families, too, were incredibly helpful in both seen and unseen ways. We really felt that there was nothing that Richard and

Cindy wouldn't do if we had a need. But many other family members were working in the background. When one of my cousins learned that Lauren had leukemia she called around to other cousins and their children to ask them to have their bone marrow tested in case Lauren needed a transplant. I have more than 30 cousins on my mother's side of the family and a number of these cousins have adult children. Many names were added to the bone marrow registry. Lauren and I found out about this long after it had been done. In one touching incident my 80+-year-old aunt, over the first winter of treatment, during the time my mom was away on holiday, called to see if there was anything she could do and that she wanted me to know, although she didn't use these actual words, that she was my mother in my mother's absence.

During this time I taught one course a term, one day a week. My dean at the university and the upper echelons of the administration had generously allowed my year-long sabbatical to be extended to two years. (I taught the courses that I was required to teach in one year over a two-year period.) By the second year of the extended sabbatical I really could have been back full-time but I didn't know that when I made the arrangements, and I am glad that I did have the time because I never felt a conflict between my responsibilities at work and my desire to care for Lauren and to put her needs first.

Each summer Lauren and I spent as much time as possible at our cottage—relaxing, gardening, reading, and swimming. Although we returned to town for treatments she had the blood count tests required before treatment at the little local hospital in cottage country. They faxed the counts to our local hospital and I would call to see if Lauren was to receive treatment or not and to arrange to come back as necessary. By the second summer, the routine was much more stable. More times than not she received her treatments on schedule. The second summer Lauren, intrepid about getting back to normal and becoming a part of her university and college, took a summer job working in the college kitchen. She worked about half-time but had to take a three-week break at one point because of a serious sunburn on the front of her feet. We had sat outside under a porch one summer morning for about an hour. Lauren's feet were bare. Usually she covered her whole body with special sun-resistant clothing and her skin with sun screen because one of the drugs that she was taking increased sun sensitivity. We thought the porch roof would protect her from the sun, but it didn't, and the resulting burn was extremely painful and kept Lauren off her feet for about three weeks.

The second year of university, after a summer working in the cafeteria, Lauren decided to live near the campus in a townhouse with a couple of other students she had met during the summer. This was a good decision as she was able to come and go to the university and meet others as she liked. She became more involved in campus life, started peer tutoring, worked on the newspaper and wrote three articles about her disease, volunteered at WPRIG (a public interest research organization), and joined the peace society and several other clubs. All of this was despite the fact that she suffered recurrent bouts of depression from the dexamethasone and ongoing fatigue and weakness. She began to try to build her strength by joining an aquatics class on campus. She walked many kilometres most days to the campus and to various activities. During this second year she continued to come home often. She needed a lot of extra support. I generally drove her to the hospital for blood tests one day and treatment the next day. I needed to be involved.

As I write Lauren is off treatment and has been for more than a year. She has had, and her family with her, the celebration of which she writes in her epilogue. She is living in a house with five other young women, planning a conference on peace and conflict for the weekend, trying to get all of her course work done before the end of term, applying for a summer work placement to work with refugees in Montreal, and just generally busily living the life of a healthy student in her third year of university.

I am back to work full-time. Life is sort of back to normal. I usually do not worry about Lauren's health. If she looks very pale, has the flu, or feels particularly tired I get alarmed, but I am usually able to put it out of my mind and trust that she is better. Although I live with uncertainty it is in the midst of optimism. I am amazed at how normal life usually seems now—when we were in the thick of it I couldn't believe in or imagine a future when Lauren's health, her well-being, could ever again be taken for granted. But then, I guess, it isn't—quite.

Lauren's Epilogue

When I look in the mirror I see a woman who is healthy. Her hair is brown and chin-length. Her skin turns rosy from walking outside in the cold. She smiles easily. This woman is new. She has risen from the ashes, come from some place where she was almost lost. Her child self had grown up, matured, and then become sick. In this illness she learned a lot about being loved and about the strength of her body. And now she is well. But what does this mean? Do 25 months of living with a life-threatening illness really matter? Why did she survive?

These questions are difficult to answer. However, they must be asked, addressed, and thought about. It would be easier to go on with my life as though nothing has changed, because in fundamental ways nothing has. I am still Lauren Nancarrow Clarke. I still have my family. I still can walk. Yet, my experience must mean something to me. So what does it mean?

Well, in a chapter (probably not even in a book, since it is so intrinsic to who I am) I cannot answer this question. I could do a lot of things with this chapter. I could tell about what it was like for me to be diagnosed, what happened at my school when I got sick and returned, how my friends dealt with my disease, and so on. However, I have chosen to use an example of a particularly special day to share some of my thoughts on my illness and on the above question of meaning.

This day was 14 November 1998, the anniversary of the end of my remission induction (1995). A few days later, 18 November, is the anniversary of my last day of chemotherapy (1997). It felt like a momentous occasion. I needed to mark it somehow—so how did I?

Throughout the course of treatment my dad had consistently asked me if I wanted to celebrate different occurrences: ending a certain drug, my remission induction day while I was still undergoing treatment, the removal of my port-a-cath. Each of these times seemed premature to me. Each time felt a little bit like we were tempting fate. I needed the security of being off of chemotherapy and feeling my body strong again before wanting to celebrate. These two things converged in November.

I wanted to have a celebration for two reasons: to thank people for their support and to show everyone that I had healed. I planned this day, along with the help of my parents, to be held at the church I attend. I wanted the location to be accessible and to feel good. I wanted it to be a place of warmth and compassion.

We were expecting 70 people.[1] Since the church easily holds more than 300, the challenge was to make the room feel comfortable for our smaller group. Mom and Marian and Dad did a wonderful job decorating and preparing the room for the day. On the morning of the celebration I was at home editing what I had written to say in front of the gathering. My parents met and worked on preparing the place. They took all morning to do this, even with the help of two of my friends. I had no idea what it was going to look like—and when I arrived I saw that there was no way that it could have been more beautiful. They had made a cosy, intimate space at the front of the room, covering walls and barriers with striking African cloths that Jess and Marian had bought while in Malawi and Zimbabwe the year before. A friend and fellow cancer patient had sent an exotic array of yellow orchids from Hawaii that sat in a place of honour. The piano was pulled over to be included in an intimate circle of chairs. The place looked smashing.

During the summer before the celebration I had spent three weeks writing poetry and creating collages and painted artwork to express some of my emotions around my illness. These pieces were on display in the main gathering area. People could look at them while entering or eating the cookies and carrots after the ceremony. My goal in producing these pieces of art was to work

---

[1] Footnoting my own epilogue? Even though we were expecting 70, we were overwhelmed by over 120 people coming to celebrate with us. Old teachers, somewhat out-of-touch friends, my nurses, and my whole extended family crowded the room. It was unbelievable.

through some of the residual sadness, anger, and confusion left from my illness. I wanted to make concrete the emotions that had only been inside of me previously. I wanted to be rid of some of these feelings. The pieces that emerged were completely different from what I had planned. Rather than simply showing anger, feelings of joy and renewal emerged. I wanted to make the negative associations towards some of the objects dissipate. I needed to 'happify' them. Thus the port-a-cath that lived in me for over two years became the centre for a flower on a painting/collage. I filled the pill bottles that had previously held 'poisons' with candies and pennies, symbolizing pleasure and luck. I was surprised at what I made, and pleased with it, too.

I felt very calm on the day. The people who were coming all loved me or knew my family well. Once they started to arrive I felt a sense of ease. This day was here and it was going to be good! Before I started to speak, two of my close women friends prayed with me about the outcome of the day. I remember we prayed for clarity of thought and that I would be able to deeply experience the day itself.

I had written the order of speaking for the day and what I was going to say. I really ran the day; however, I could not have done this without the absolute backing of my family. They created the food and the space that everyone enjoyed. They gave me the peace of mind to be able to be fully present in what I was saying and doing. The day was a wonderful way for me to say, 'Hey, I'm back and I'm ready to dance with life again!' I had energy to organize and visualize the day and pull it off—what a joy!

I started the time by thanking people. I wanted to express gratitude to everyone; however, this is a monumental task. How to thank the uncle who carried my bed up and down stairs every day so that I could be in the common room with others? How to thank the friends who made dinner for my mom and me every Tuesday for a school term when I was first diagnosed? How to show thanks to the people who love me and would do anything in their power for me? I asked different groups of people to stand separately and I expressed thanks to them, listing some of the specific things that I could remember people doing, the special kindnesses they had

Baseball

Remember when
you called 'move in'
    and they did?
I recognized
not some silly sexist remark
but the   truth.
    (weak, sick,
    grounded)
And so they did
and so I hit.

I would like to say
it   flew,
        past the spruce that lined the field,
            over Rob, over Aaron, over Shannon
it sailed to the   farthest
region of the diamond.

It didn't.

It landed at your pitcher's feet.
Someone else,
I'm not sure who,
substituted and ran to first base.

I pretended
to smile
    sit back,
        wait,
until I could show
you
    me
        again.

shown. I wanted publicly to acknowledge my parents' supporters, my friends, my teachers, my medical care team, my extended and immediate family. My parents and sister were the hardest individuals to thank. Afterwards, I came to the conclusion that my thank-you to my immediate family was the fact that I am alive. It is as simple as that.

I went on to talk about how I saw my recovery as a miracle. I said that this miracle was given to me by God. This miracle was given to me by those who had supported me physically, emotionally, and spiritually. The miracle is mine because my body was able to take the chemotherapy and come out all right. Medicine, the drugs that so ravished me, is part of this miracle. The vitamin C and also the therapeutic touch treatments my mom and stepmom gave me are part of it. My aquafit classes have helped. My family supported this miracle. My walks to school aided in creating it. My friends helped by letting me digest my experiences and keeping me laughing. Through all of this a miracle was created.

This miracle meant that I could celebrate my recovery and wellness with everyone. Traditionally, the only times we get together to celebrate significantly are marriages, major anniversaries, and birthdays. However, we also gather for funerals. As one of my high school teachers commented jokingly, this day was a 'non-funeral'. It is true: the alternative outcome of the disease I had is death. But I feel it is as important to mark life as it is to mark its passing. This celebration was an affirmation of life.

On the celebration day I tried to respond and deal with the questions of 'How has cancer changed your life?' and 'How have you grown?' These types of questions are the ones that most people ask me now that it is all done. On the one hand, I would like to have an easy answer to give people. This would help both them and me. I can think of some things. However, my core rebels against the thought that I needed cancer to 'wake me up' or to make me 'slow down'. We tend to impose this belief system on people, but it is not fully true. We need to know that the ending is 'happily ever after', that the worry and fear we held about the person is no longer necessary and that everything turned out 'for the best'. My heart fights this because it makes me feel criticized and demeaned—it implies

> **word**
>
> Call it by name:
> cancer
>   leukemia
>   sick
> diagnosed.
>
> As if labelled, named,
> by speaking   incessantly
> it might be
> overpowered, destroyed,
>
>   regain my strength.
>
> Words
> language itself,
> numb.
>
> For a word does not
>   throw up every day at three,
>   cry as hair clumps in front,
>   believe that being held can save.
>
> A word does not
>   cure.

that I needed improvement. Also, it feels as if the disease, and not my response to the disease, has made me a stronger ('better'?) person.

Yet, I would think that one of my learnings is that I am powerless in most matters in my life. I can perhaps control my emotions, with meditation and if I am in full capacity of them. But what else can I 'control'? I should know that there are much larger powers than me working out the world's existence. However, I still do believe that it is not the illness but our response that creates a change in us. So should people ask me 'How has your response to your illness changed you?' Perhaps. But it does sound a little convoluted.

In response to this unasked question (on that day) I chose to identify three blessings in my life: the people around me, my physical being, and my newly developing belief in a Creator. I knew before I became ill that people loved me, but when a difficult thing happens it seems to free us up to show each other how much we really care. When I was first diagnosed, my hospital room was a garden of roses, mums, birds of paradise, and carnations. My wall was covered with dozens of cards expressing people's feelings over my illness. My homeroom class at the time sent me a pictorial account of their lives, telling me how much I was missed. People were constantly calling and asking what they could do to be of help. Some people did not know what to say, but they called or sent a card anyway. My aunts and uncles cared for me and my parents in a way that I so hope to emulate in my life. My support circle (including those people who primarily supported my family) is huge! My illness allowed people to care unashamedly for me and my family.

During the celebration I did not talk to the assembled group about those friends who had disappointed me. Some of these friends did not know what to say to me and so said nothing. One whom I wanted to rely on was dealing with her own challenges and could not give as much as I needed. And no one else had cancer. The first year and a half was a lonely time. I left high school and entered university. I walked the paths at my university in a vague discontent of isolation. I had cancer—practically no one knew, and those few who did could not comprehend what it meant to me. During my illness it was not fear but loneliness that caused most of my tears.

The second blessing I have recognized is my sense of my physical strength. Before I was sick, my body was never important to me. It did what I needed it to do but nothing more than that. I did not know the joy of exercise. I did not know how it feels to have run a block and be more alive than ever before. I did not know that jumping is a miracle. When I was the sickest I had trouble walking by myself because of nausea. Later, my decreased muscle strength held

> **untitled**
>
> A hardness
> slowly swallows what's left.
>   I cry out to stop it,
> I fear that if I don't
> something else might.
>
> Something else
> that could be
>   the end.
>
> They say you can only cry for so long—
> until you must
>   straighten up,
>   look ahead,
>   think clearly.
>
> If not
> I might be left alone
>   afraid
> feeling nothing but a hardness
>
> in my chest.

me back. I needed to stop at the bottom of a set of stairs in order to climb them. I would first decide how to best go up them, often with help from another or from my hand, and then I would slowly make my way to the top. I now revel in jumping, dancing, running. I can bike once again! I love swimming laps and doing aquafitness classes. My body works for me and it gives me so much joy.

    The final growth (blessing) is my developing faith. I cannot say clearly where it is going or where it will end up, but I am on the journey. I grew up in an Anglican church to which I never truly connected. However, now I feel that I am choosing my faith. I am attending chapel services weekly at my college and this gives me a good resource to bounce my beliefs off of and to be challenged. I also attend Rockway Mennonite Church, which is led by a wonderful pastor who did the concluding blessing at my celebration. But my faith has more to do with the spirit that floods my body and the natural world around me at this time than it does with any particular figure. I do see God beside me, holding my hand, walking with me, guiding my feet, and healing my body. The Creator is present always and I feel God's presence in my prayers.

These are the things that I identified at the celebration as being major gifts. I would like to add that I also try to make more decisions based on my health and stress level than I did before. (Still, with my new-found strength it is hard to choose sleeping over dancing!) This celebration was a wonderful way for me to thank and to celebrate. I know people who came enjoyed it. As my former debating coach and mentor, Jim Weber, said, 'Lauren, you are doing something which it would be well for all of us to do. You are pausing for a moment of thanksgiving, for a moment of reflection, a stocktaking, a meditation on meaning. You've drawn together a community of people who know you and care about you and who will be enriched by being present.'

Yet, I am still trying to make sense of what happened. Most of the time it is distant. I have come through cancer and I am now well. But it is not that simple. I forget now that I had cancer. I forget the pain, the fear, the effort, the loneliness. I forget what happened to me. Recently I forgot to call to make an appointment to go to the hospital for my regular blood work. Just like that, what once was my world is no longer. Chemotherapy, its impact on my immune system, and the fear of catching something serious from someone are gone. There are small reminders: my need for naps every day, my more easily bruised body, my shortish hair. But these are minor things. I feel well. I am eating more healthily, exercising regularly, and trying to choose an activity level that does not give me too much stress. Yet, there are times when the enormity of what I have been through overtakes me. Sometimes I am overcome with tears and grief. I want two years of my life to mean something—I want every day to mean something. Somehow I need to come to a

The Bubble

I heard about a boy in a bubble.
Immortalized by Paul Simon.
Deified by medical establishments.
The boy so sheltered, so protected,
he never felt his mother's hand,
living away
    tucked away
        stuck away
            so he would live another day,
alone, pure, empty.

I say to him
(was it Robert? Steven? Doug?)
that I understand a drop
of how you feel.
I know a tear of what
you know.

Because I lived in a room,
blocked off,
that held a warning sign.
A room where you were masked,
gloved, dehumanized
to enter.

You stood, coughing, outside
waving through the window
to show me your love
waving
through too thick glass

So again I say to him
(was it Billy? Chris? Matt?)
I understand a drop,
    I know a tear.

conclusion with this illness, but I think that this conclusion may still be years and learnings away. I know that I am healthier now than I was before I became ill. I also know that being true to myself is the only way to make myself and others happy. I know, too, that life is not about the absence of pain but rather about dealing with every situation with as much grace and love as possible. So, what will the next years bring me? I do not know, but I do know that I am loving life and anticipating the coming years with much enthusiasm. I feel so well.

I have gone through a lot and I am healthy. But we all go through 'a lot' and we all need to be healthy. I hope that you will hold a celebration for yourself, too—not because of leukemia or another illness, but simply because you are alive and unique.

Peace on your journey,

LAUREN

BIBLIOGRAPHY

Adams, David W. 1992. *Parents of Children with Cancer Speak Out: Problems, Needs and Sources of Help*. Toronto: Candlelighters Childhood Cancer Foundation.

Anderson, E., and P. Anderson. 1987. 'General practitioners and alternative medicine', *Journal of the Royal College of General Practitioners* 37: 52-5.

Armstrong, Pat, and Hugh Armstrong. 1996. *Wasting Away: The Undermining of Canadian Health Care*. Toronto: Oxford University Press.

Balter, Michael. 1995. 'Cheronbyl's thyroid cancer toll', *Science* 270, 15: 1785-9.

Barbarin, Oscar A. 1987. 'Psychosocial risks and vulnerability: A review of the theoretical and empirical bases of preventative family focused services for survivors of childhood cancer', *Journal of Psychosocial Oncology* 5, 4: 25-41.

_____ and Mark A. Chesler. 1984. 'Coping as interpersonal strategy: families with childhood cancer', *Family Systems Medicine* 2, 3: 279-89.

_____ and _____. 1986. 'The medical context of parental coping with childhood cancer', *American Journal of Community Psychology* 14, 2 (Apr.): 221-35.

_____, D. Hughes, and M. Chesler. 1985. 'Stress, coping and marital functioning among parents of children with cancer', *Journal of Marriage and the Family* 47: 473-80.

Bard, M., and R.D. Dyk. 1956. 'The psychodynamic significance of beliefs regarding the cause of serious illness', *Psychoanalytic Review* 43: 146-62.

Barr, Ronald D., William Furlong, John R. Horseman, David Feeny, George W. Torrance, and Sheila Weitzman. 1996. 'The monetary costs of childhood cancer to the families of patients', *International Journal of Oncology* 8: 933-40.

Bearison, David J. 1991. *They Never Want to Tell You: Children Talk about Cancer*. Cambridge, Mass.: Harvard University Press.

_____, Andrea J. Sadow, Linda Granowetter, and Gary Winkel. 1993. 'Patients' and parents' causal attributions for childhood cancer', *Journal of Psychosocial Oncology* 11, 13: 47-61.

Benson, Herbert. 1979. *The Mind-Body Effect*. New York: Simon & Schuster.

Birenbaum, Linda K. 1990. 'Family coping with childhood cancer', *Hospice Journal* 6, 3: 17-33.

Bluebond-Langer, Myra. 1978. *The Private Worlds of Dying Children*. Princeton, NJ: Princeton University Press.

Brown, Phil. 1995. 'Naming and framing: The social construction of diagnosis

and illness', *Journal of Health and Social Behavior* 33: 267-78.
Broyard, A. 1992. *Intoxicated by My Illness*. New York: Clarison Potler Publishers.
Bueckert, Dennis. 1998. 'Children receiving too many antibiotics for ear infections: study', *Kitchener-Waterloo Record*, 3 June.
Cassileth, B.R., E.J. Lusk, T.B. Strouse, and B.J. Bodenheimer. 1984. 'Contemporary unorthodox treatments in cancer medicine', *Annals of Internal Medicine* 101: 105-12.
Caudell, Kathryn Ann. 1996. 'Psychoneuroimmunology and innovative behavioral intervention in patients with leukemia', *Oncology Nursing Forum* 23, 3: 493-502.
Chesler, Mark A., and Oscar A. Barbarin. 1984. 'Difficulties of Providing Help in a Crisis: Relationships between Parents of Children with Cancer and Their Friends', *Journal of Social Issues* 40, 4: 113-34.
_____ and _____. 1987. *Childhood Cancer and the Family: Meeting the Challenge of Stress and Support*. New York: Brunner/Mazel.
Chopra, Deepak. 1989. *Quantum Healing: Exploring the Frontiers of Body Medicine*. New York: Bantam Books.
Chow, Wong-Ho, Martha S. Linet, Jonathan M. Liff, and Raymond S. Greenberg. 1996. 'Cancers in children', in David Scotlenfeld and Joseph Frauneri Jr, eds, *Cancer Epidemiology and Prevention*, 2nd edn. New York: Oxford University Press.
Clark, Jack A., Deborah A. Potter, and John B. McKinlay. 1991. 'Bringing social structure back into clinical decision-making', *Social Science and Medicine* 32, 8: 853-63.
Clarke, Juanne Nancarrow. 1985. *It's Cancer: The Personal Experiences of Women Who Have Received Cancer Diagnosis*. Toronto: IPI.
_____. 1992. 'Cancer, heart disease and AIDS: What do the media tell us about these diseases?', *Health Communication* 4, 2: 105-20.
_____. 1996. *Health, Illness, and Medicine in Canada*, 2nd edn. Toronto: Oxford University Press.
Cockerham, W.C. 1989. *Medical Sociology*, 4th edn. Englewood Cliffs, NJ: Prentice-Hall.
Colburn, Theo, D. Dumanoski, and J.P. Myers. 1996. *Our Stolen Future*. New York: Penguin.
Corelli, R. 1997. 'The Charity Industry', *Maclean's* (15 Sept.): 68-72.
Cousins, Norman. 1979. *Anatomy of an Illness as Perceived by the Patient*. Toronto: Bantam Books.
Delvaux, Nicole, Darius Razavi, and Christine Farvacques. 1988. 'Cancer care: A stress for health professionals', *Social Science and Medicine* 27, 2: 159-66.
Desmeules, Marie. 1995. 'The Canadian childhood cancer control programme', *Contact* 7, 1: 1-3.
Dossey, Larry. 1993. *Healing Wounds: The Power of Prayer and the Practice of Medicine*. San Francisco: Harper.
_____. 1996. *Prayer is Good Medicine*. San Francisco: Harper.
_____. 1997. *Be Careful What You Pray For*. San Francisco: Harper.
Downer, S.M., M.M. Cody, P. McCluskey, P.D. Wilson, S.J. Arnott, T.A. Lister, and M.L. Slevin. 1994. 'Pursuit and practice of complementary therapies by can-

cer patients receiving conventional treatment', *British Medical Journal* 309: 86-9.
Eisenberg, David M., et al. 1993. 'Unconventional medicine in the United States—Prevalence, costs, and patterns of use', *New England Journal of Medicine* 328, 4: 246-52.
Eiser, C., T. Havermans, and J.R. Eiser. 1995. 'Parents' attributions about childhood cancer: Implications for relationships with medical staff', *Child-Care, Health and Development* 21, 1 (Jan.): 31-42.
Epp, Jake. 1986. *Achieving Health for All: A Framework for Health Promotion*. Ottawa. Minister of National Health and Welfare.
Epstein, Samuel. 1979. *The Politics of Cancer*. Garden City, NY: Anchor Books.
_____. 1998. *The Politics of Cancer Revisited*. Fremont Center, NY: East Ridge Press.
Evans-Emery, Janet. 1993. 'Perceived source of stress among pediatric oncology nurses', *Journal of Pediatric Oncology Nursing* 10, 3: 87-92.
Fife, B., J. Norton, and G. Groom. 1987. 'The family's adaptation to childhood leukemia', *Social Science and Medicine* 24: 159-68.
Freudenberger, Herbert J. 1974. 'Staff burn-out', *Journal of Social Issues* 30, 1: 159-65.
Goldszmidt, M., C. Levitt, E. Duatre-Franco, and J. Kaczorowski. 1995. 'Complementary health care services: A survey of general practitioners' views', *Canadian Medical Association Journal* 153, 1: 29-35.
Haas, Jack, and William Shaffir. 1977a. 'The Professionalization of Medical Students: Developing Competence and a Cloak of Competence', *Symbolic Interaction* 1: 71-88.
_____ and _____. 1977b. *Becoming Doctors: The Adoption of a Cloak of Competence*. Greenwich, Conn.: JAI.
Hadley, C.M. 1988. 'Complementary medicine and the general practitioner: A survey of general practitioners in the Wellington area', *New Zealand Medical Journal* 101: 766-8.
Hafferty, Frederick W. 1988. 'Cadaver stories and the emotional socialization of medical students', *Journal of Health and Social Behavior* 29 (Dec.): 344-56.
Hall, A.M., T. Knighton, P. Reed, P. Busiere, D. McRae, and P. Owen. 1998. *Caring Canadians, Involved Canadians: Highlights from 1997 National Survey of Giving, Volunteering and Participating*. Statistics Canada, Cat. no. 71-542-XPE. Ottawa: Ministry of Industry.
Hochschild, Arlie Russell. 1979. 'Emotion work, feeling rules, and social structure', *American Journal of Sociology* 85, 3: 551-75.
_____. 1983. *The Managed Heart: Commercialization of Human Feeling*. Berkeley: University of California Press.
Horowitz, Sala. 1998. 'The power of more than one', *Alternative and Complementary Therapies* (Apr.): 84-7.
Hughes, Patricia M., and Stuart Lieberman. 1990. 'Troubled parents' vulnerability and stress in childhood cancer', *British Journal of Medical Psychology* 63, 1 (Mar.): 53-64.
Hutchcroft, S., A. Clarke, Y. Mao, M. Desmeules, D. Dryer, M. Hodges, J.M. Leclerc, M. McBride, W. Pelletier, and R. Yanosky. 1996. *This Battle Which I Must Fight:*

Cancer in Canada's Children and Teenagers. Ottawa: Supply and Services Canada.
IMS Health Strategic Technologies. 1999. 'Doctors Practising in Canada', data on file. Toronto.
Kalnins, I.V., M.P. Churchill, and G.E. Terry. 1980. 'Concurrent stresses in families with a leukemic child', *Journal of Pediatric Psychology* 5: 81-92.
Kazak, Anne E., and Ginnette S. Nachman. 1991. 'Family research on childhood chronic illness: Pediatric oncology as an example', *Journal of Family Psychology* 4, 4 (June): 462-83.
Keene, Nancy. 1997. *Childhood Leukemia: A Guide For Families, Friends and Caregivers*. Cambridge, Mass.: O'Reilly.
Kirkpatrick, J., I. Hoffman, and E. Futterman. 1974. 'Dilemma of trust: Relationship between medical caregivers and parents of fatally ill children', *Pediatrics* 54: 169-75.
Klein, Bonnie S. 1997. *Slow Dance: A Story of Stroke, Love and Disability*. Toronto: Vintage Canada.
Klein, Michael C. 1997. 'Too close for comfort', *Canadian Medical Association Journal* 156, 1: 53-5.
Kleinman, Arthur. 1988. *The Illness Narratives: Suffering, Healing and the Human Condition*. New York: Basic Books.
Kupst, M.J., J.L. Schulman, G. Honig, H. Maurer, E. Morgan, and D. Fochtman. 1982. 'Family coping with childhood leukemia: one year after diagnosis', *Journal of Pediatric Psychology* 7: 157-74.
Lalonde, Marc. 1974. *A New Perspective on the Health of Canadians*. Ottawa. Information Canada.
LaValley, J. William, and M.J. Verhoef. 1995. 'Integrating complementary medicine and health care services into practice', *Canadian Medical Association Journal* 153, 1: 45-9.
Lazarus, R.S. 1966. *Psychological Stress and the Coping Process*. New York: McGraw-Hill.
Lerner, Michael. 1994. *Choices in Healing: Integrating the Best of Conventional and Complementary Approaches to Cancer*. Cambridge, Mass.: MIT Press.
Lerner, M.J., and C.H. Simmons. 1966. 'Observers' reaction to the "innocent victim": Compassion or rejection?', *Journal of Personality and Social Psychology* 5: 319-25.
LeShan, Lawrence. 1977. *You Can Fight For Your Life: Emotional Factors in the Causation of Cancer*. New York: M. Evans & Company.
Lozowski, Sheryl, Mark A. Chesler, and Barbara K. Chesney. 1993. 'Parental intervention in the medical care of children with cancer', *Journal of Psychosocial Oncology* 11, 3: 63-88.
McBride, Mary L. 1998. 'Childhood cancer and environmental contaminants', *Canadian Journal of Public Health* 89, 1: S53-S62.
Maguire, G.P. 1983. 'The psychological sequelae of childhood leukemia', in W. Duncan, ed., *Pediatric Oncology*. Berlin: Springer-Verlag, 47-56.
Martinson, Ida M., and Marsha H. Cohen. 1988. 'Themes from a longitudinal study of family reaction to childhood cancer', *Journal of Psychosocial Oncology* 6, 3-4: 81-98.

Maslach, C., and S. Jackson. 1986. *Maslach Burnout Inventory*. Palo Alto, Calif.: Consulting Psychologists Press.
Mattson, A. 1979. 'Long-term physical illness in childhood: A challenge to psychosocial adaptation', in C. Garfield, ed, *Stress and Survival*. St Louis: C.V. Mosby, 253-63.
Millman, Marcia. 1977. *The Unkindest Cut*. New York: William Morrow.
Nelson, Melvin D. 1992. 'Socio-economic status and childhood mortality in North Carolina', *American Journal of Public Health* 82, 8: 1131-3.
Overholser, James C., and Gregory K. Fritz. 1990. 'The impact of childhood cancer on the family', *Journal of Psychosocial Oncology* 8, 4: 71-85.
Parsons, Talcott. 1954. 'The professions and the social structure', in *Essays in Sociological Theory*. Glencoe, Ill.: Free Press, 428-47.
Pilnick, Alison. 1998. '"Why didn't you just say that?" Dealing with issues of symmetry, knowledge and competence in the pharmicist/client encounter', *Sociology of Health and Illness* 20, 1: 29-51.
Ramirez, A.J., J. Graham, M.A. Richards, A. Cull, W.M. Gregory, M.S. Leaning, and D.C. Snashall. 1995. 'Burnout and psychiatric disorder among cancer clinicians', *British Journal of Cancer* 71, 6: 1263-9.
Reilly, D.T. 1983. 'Young doctors' views on alternative medicine', *British Medical Journal* 287: 337-9.
Rolland, J. 1984. 'Towards a psychosocial typology of chronic and life-threatening illness', *Family Systems Medicine* 2: 245-62.
_____. 1987. 'Chronic illness and the life cycle: a conceptual framework', *Family Process* 26: 203-21.
Ruccione, Kathleen S., Mary Waskerwitz, Jonathan Buckley, Gail Perrin, and G. Denman Hammond. 1994. 'What caused my child's cancer? Parents' responses to an epidemiology study of childhood cancer', *Journal of Pediatric Oncology Nursing* 11, 2: 71-84.
Schachter, L., B.M. Weingarten, and E.E. Kahan. 1993. 'Attitudes of family physicians to nonconventional therapies: A challenge to science as the basis of therapeutics', *Archives of Family Medicine* 2: 1268-70.
Schutz, Alfred. 1967. *The Problem of Social Reality*. Collected Papers 1. The Hague: Martinus Nijhoff.
Siegal, Bernie. 1986. *Love, Medicine and Miracles: Lessons Learned about Self-healing from a Surgeon's Experience*. New York: Harper & Row.
Simonton, O. Carl, Stephanie Mathews-Simonton, and James L. Creighton. 1978. *Getting Well Again*. Toronto: Bantam Books.
Smith, Allen C., and Sherryl Kleinman. 1989. 'Managing emotions in medical school: Students' contacts with the living and the dead', *Social Psychology Quarterly* 52, 1: 56-69.
Sontag, Susan. 1979. *Illness as Metaphor*. New York: Vintage Books.
Spiegal, David. 1991. 'A Psychosocial Intervention and Survival Time of Patients with Metastatic Breast Cancer', *Advances* 7, 3: 10-19.
Stahley, Geraldine Butts. 1988. 'Psychosocial aspects of the stigma of cancer: An overview', *Journal of Psychosocial Oncology* 6, 3-4: 3-27.
Statistics Canada. 1997. *Cancer Incidence in Canada, 1969-1993*. Ottawa: Statistics Canada.
Steingraber, Sandra. 1997. *Living Downstream*. Reading, Mass.: Addison-Wesley.

Stern, Marilyn, and Edward Arenson. 1989. 'Childhood cancer stereotype: Impact on adult perceptions of children', *Journal of Pediatric Psychology* 14, 4 (Dec.): 593-605.

―――, Susan Ross, and Mary Beilass. 1991.'Medical students' perceptions of children: Modifying a childhood cancer stereotype', *Journal of Pediatric Psychology* 16, 1 (Feb.): 27-38.

Stewart, W. 1996. *The Charity Game: Greed, Waste and Fraud in Canada's $86 Billion a Year Compassion Industry*. Vancouver: Douglas & McIntyre.

Sudnow, David. 1967. *Passing on the Social Organization of Dying*. Englewood Cliffs, NJ: Prentice-Hall.

Taylor, Shelley. 1983.'Adjustment to threatening events: A theory of cognitive adaptation', *American Psychology* 38: 1161-3.

Todd, A.D. 1994. *Double Vision: An East-West Collaboration for Coping with Cancer*. Middletown, Conn.: Wesleyan University Press.

Torrance, George M. 1998.'Hospitals as health factories', in David Coburn, Carl D'Arcy, and George M. Torrance, eds, *Health and Canadian Society*, 3rd edn. Toronto: University of Toronto Press.

Tully, Patricia, and Etienne Saint-Pierre. 1997.'Downsizing Canada's hospitals, 1986/1987 to 1994/1995', *Health Reports* 8, 4 (Spring): 33-40.

Van Dongen-Melman, J.E., J.F.A. Pruyn, G.E. Van Zanen, and J.A.R. Sanders-Woudstra. 1986.'Coping with childhood cancer: A conceptual view', *Journal of Psychosocial Oncology* 41, 2: 147-61.

――― and J.A. Sanders-Woudstra. 1986. 'Psychosocial aspects of childhood cancer: A review of the literature', *Journal of Child Psychology and Psychiatry and Allied Disciplines* 27, 2 (Mar.): 145-80.

Verhoef, M.J., and L.R. Sutherland. 1995.'Alternative medicine and general practitioners', *Canadian Family Physician* 41: 1005.

Wager, Susan. 1996. *A Doctor's Guide to Therapeutic Touch*. New York: Penguin.

Waitzkin, Howard. 1989. 'Medicine superstructure and microplitics', *Social Science and Medicine* 13A: 601-9.

Wharton, R., and G. Lewith. 1986.'Complementary medicine and the general practitioner', *British Medical Journal* 92: 1498-500.

Whippen, Deborah A., and George P. Canellos. 1991.'Burnout syndrome in the practice of oncology: Results of a random survey of 1,000 oncologists', *Journal of Clinical Oncology* 9, 10: 1916-20.

Wong-Wylie, Gina, and Ronne F. Jevne. 1997.'Patient hope: Exploring the interactions between physicians and HIV seropositive individuals', *Qualitative Health Research* 7, 1: 32-56.

Yates, P.M., G. Beadle, A. Clavarino, J.M. Najman, D. Thomson, G. Williams, L. Kenny, S. Roberts, B. Mason, and D. Schlect. 1993.'Patients with terminal cancer who use alternative therapies: their beliefs and practices', *Sociology of Health and Illness* 15: 199.

APPENDIX

RESOURCES FOR CHILDHOOD CANCER

BOOK AND LIBRARY RESOURCES

There are two books dealing with childhood leukemia, one for children and young people and the other for adults, that I highly recommend. Each provides an overview of the characteristics of and the treatment for leukemia today. With chapter headings such as 'You' and subheadings such as 'your body', 'your blood and leukemia', 'one day at a time', and 'treatments' (things you wanted to know, but didn't think you would understand), as well as many diagrams, *You and Leukemia: A Day at a Time* (Philadelphia: W.B. Saunders, 1988), by Dr Lynn S. Baker, is a valuable resource for parents and children to have on hand over the course of treatment. The other, *Childhood Leukemia: A Guide for Families, Friends and Caregivers* (Cambridge, Mass.: O'Reilly, 1997), is written by Nancy Keene, the mother of a child who had leukemia and a writer who has developed the O'Reilly Patient-Centered Guide health series to empower patients and their families. This book includes medical and psychosocial information, as well as insights into how various children and parents have experienced leukemia via selections from interviews that are interspersed throughout. Chapter headings include: Diagnosis, What Is Leukemia, Coping with Procedure, What Is a Clinical Trial, Family and Friends, Forming a Partnership with the Medical Team, Surviving Your Child's Hospitalization, Choosing a Catheter, Sources of Support, Chemotherapy, Common Side Effects of Chemotherapy, Radiation, Record Keeping and Finances, Nutrition, School, Siblings, Feelings, Communication and Behaviour, End of Treatment and Beyond, Relapse, Bone Marrow Transplantation, and Death and Bereavement. The book also has five appendices. It is a positive, practical, and informed resource for parents.

In addition, Candlelighters, the national foundation for childhood cancer in Canada, has available an annotated resource catalogue listing over 300 books, pamphlets, and videos on childhood cancer, its treatment, the long-term effects and side-effects of treatment, and methods for control of symptoms. It also includes psychosocial and educational resources on such topics as coping, school re-entry, siblings, and bereavement. The guide comes with an order form and price list.

Many public and university libraries allow access to the latest medical, scientific, epidemiological, and socio-psychological literature from around the world. Most highly respected journals are listed and annotated on databases, available on CD-Rom format. It is possible to use searches that are specific to the field, such as Medline (medical research and epidemiology), Psychlit (psychological literature), and Sociofile (sociological resources).

CHILDHOOD CANCER WEB SITES

Treatment Protocol Groups

The Pediatric Oncology Group
The Pediatric Oncology Group is a National Cancer Institute-sponsored clinical trials co-operative group. The focus of this US-based research group is controlling childhood cancer.
http://www.pog.ufl.edu/

The Children's Cancer Group
The Children's Cancer Group is a national co-operative research organization in the US devoted to developing new treatments and cures for cancers of children and young adults. The group is a partner with the National Childhood Cancer Foundation.
http:www.nccf.org/nccf/ccg_who.htm

Medical and Government Health Organization Sites

University of Pennsylvania Cancer Centre
Pediatric oncology information with discussion groups on clinical trials, meds, coping; information on bone marrow transplants, research, and study reports. Also provides survivor stories, support group discussion, and access to their newsletter.
http://cancer.med.upenn.edu/

National Cancer Institute
Information is divided for patient, health professional, and basic researcher. Provides information on treatments, screening, prevention, and genetics. Offers support and information on clinical trials.
http://cancernet.nci.nih.gov/

University of Colorado Pediatric Resource Center
This site offers information on diseases, treatments, cancer family issues, activism. It also has information on other organizations, books, and other resources.
http://www.acor.org/

Information and Support Group Sites

Children's Cancer Web
Offers an international guide to Internet resources for childhood cancer.
http://www.ncl.ac.uk/~nch.www/guide/guide2htm

Childhood Leukemia Center
Adapted from *Childhood Leukemia: A Guide for Families, Friends and Caregivers* by Nancy Keene. Includes information for parents on coping, keeping track of blood counts, and helpful organizations.
http://www.acor.org/nkeene/

Cancer Guide by Steve Dunn
Straightforward information on confronting statistics, stories from patients, a guide to clinical trials, and how to research the literature. Also offers information on alternative medicine.
http://cancerguide.org/tour.html

Families with Children with Cancer
Provides information on the organization's offerings of support, projects and events, and advocacy. Includes their newsletter, as well as library resources and information for the newly diagnosed and other Internet resources.
http://www.interlog.com/~fcc/

Candlelighters Foundation
Provides information on the organization. A resource site with information on various cancers and issues, such as siblings and coping.
http://www.candlelighters.ca/

Leukemia Busters
British-based organization whose objective is to raise money to fund research to fight leukemia.
http://www.penlex.org.uk/

Starbright
Starbright creates projects for seriously ill children and teens to address their challenges and their questions. The organization offers videos for teens on coping and strategies on being in the hospital, as well as health-care information in terms children can understand.
http://www.starbright.org/

National Childhood Cancer Foundation
NCCF is a non-profit organization that supports pediatric cancer treatment and research projects in the US, Canada, and Australia. This network of pediatric specialists is called the Children's Cancer Group. The site offers stories, information on clinical trials, and facts on childhood cancer.
http://www.nccf.org/

Cancer Kids
Cancer Kids helps kids with cancer tell their stories.
http://www.cancerkids.org/

Dalhousie University
Offers booklets for parents to help their children understand pain.
http://is.dal.ca/~pedpain/selfhp.html/

Personal Pages

The Never Ending Squirrel Tale Web Site
This site has practical tips and encouragement for the parents of kids with cancer. It is written by parents.
http://www.squirreltales.com/

BandAides and Blackboards
Helps kids with medical problems when they return to school. Deals with teasing and other relevant issues.
http://funrsc.fairfield.edu/

Jeffrey's Folks Cancer Link
This is a support group for families touched by childhood cancer.
http://www.escape.ca/~douglas/cancer.html

Melinda's Home Page
Young girl with cancer provides information on cancer resources.
Http://www.monkeyboy.com/melinda/

Health System Organizations

Government/Research

Pediatric Oncology Group of Ontario

POGO, established in 1983, is an organization funded by the Ministry of Health. The organization is comprised of professionals, including pediatric oncologists, nurses, psychologists, social workers, child life specialists, pharmacists, nutritionists, data managers, dentists, and others who volunteer their time to be a voice for childhood cancer. POGO has created the Centre for Comprehensive Research on Childhood Cancer to undertake research activity; it maintains a database to analyse the demand for services and trends. POGO also implemented a networked information system, POGONIS, as a provincial information resource on childhood cancer.

Pediatric Oncology Group of Ontario
620 University Avenue
Suite 702
Toronto, Ontario M5G 2C1

telephone: (416) 592-1232
fax: (416) 592-1285

Consumer and Advocacy Groups

Candlelighters: Childhood Cancer Foundation Canada

Candlelighters is a national organization founded in 1987. When it began the organization was funded completely by the Canadian Cancer Society. The CCS no longer provides funding, though Candlelighters and the CCS maintain a working relationship. It is now funded through private and public donations, grants, and corporate sponsorships. Pizza Hut Canada is the national corporate sponsor of Candlelighters. There are provincial directors in each province who are parent volunteers. Candlelighters' objectives are to provide education, advocacy, and support to families of children with cancer. Candlelighters offers a 'Touch the Sky' kit designed for children aged 5 to 12 and their parents. The kit provides a stuffed lion and a tape recording for children to help them understand their illness, as well as a manual for parents to help them cope with their child's illness. Candlelighters presently distributes 1,500 kits a year. The organization offers a Family Assistance Program to assist families with the added financial burdens for expenses related to their child's cancer. A 'Back to School' program is presently being developed to assist the child, teachers, and fellow students with the specific difficulties and challenges of returning to school. *Contact* is a quarterly newsletter printed and distributed by the Candlelighters Foundation that offers current health and medical information, personal testimonies, and new resources for the reader. This organization is also working towards an active network for teens.

Candlelighters: Childhood Cancer Foundation Canada
55 Eglinton Avenue East, Suite 401   telephone: 1-800-363-1062
Toronto, Ontario M4P 1G8   (416) 489-6440
   fax: (416) 489-9812

Interlink Community Cancer Nurses Paediatric Programme
Interlink began with one nurse funded by the Hospital for Sick Children in Toronto. An additional four nurses have been added to the program as a result of assistance from Candlelighters Canada and a grant from the Trillium Foundation of Ontario. Interlink is modelled after MacMillan Nurses in the United Kingdom. The nurses work closely with families, helping them cope with cancer, and act as a link between family, hospital, and community. They assist the family in the transition from hospital to home. They serve as the liaison with the child's school, assisting all parties, including siblings, in the adjustment. Their future goal is to implement this program in all provinces.

Interlink Community Cancer Nurses
620 University Avenue, 7th Floor,   telephone: (416) 599-5465
Toronto, Ontario, M5G 2C2   fax: (416) 599-5972

The Children's Wish Foundation
The Children's Wish Foundation is a non-profit organization established in 1984. Currently there are chapters in all provinces. The foundation relies on donations from corporations, individuals, and its own fund-raising efforts. The goal is to grant wishes to children with high-risk, life-threatening illnesses. Children aged 3 to 18 years are eligible. The child must be referred, but referrals may come from anyone with an interest. Medical forms must be presented for approval.

The Children's Wish Foundation of Canada
1730 McPherson Court, Unit 30   telephone: (905) 831-9474
Pickering, Ontario, L1W 3E6   1-800-267-9474
   fax: (905) 831-2244
   e-mail: cwf_ontario@compuserve.com

Ronald McDonald House
Ronald McDonald House is a national organization established in 1981. Today there are 10 independently operated houses across Canada. The houses are initially started with funding from McDonald's Restaurants of Canada, then continue to operate on their own. They operate through corporate sponsorship and their own fund-raising. Although not officially affiliated, they do work closely with hospitals since they are geographically situated to service people in need of hospital care. Ronald McDonald houses are homes away from home for out-of-town families whose children are receiving hospital treatment for cancer or other major pediatric illnesses. Families are charged a nominal fee

for accommodation.

Ronald McDonald House
26 Gerrard St. East telephone: (416) 977-1458
Toronto, Ontario, M5B 1G3 fax: (416) 977-8807

Families with Children with Cancer
Families with Children with Cancer is a group established in the province of Ontario in 1985 and is an affiliate of Candlelighters Canada. It consists of 20 support groups, which are run independently. This is a non-profit organization relying on donations. Its goal is to provide support, education, and advocacy to families. Future projects include developing a music therapy program and developing a bereavement and support program with the assistance of an occupational therapist.

Families with Children with Cancer c/o Georgia Bowen
46 Hogarth Avenue telephone: (416) 465-5157
Toronto, Ontario M4K 1K1 http://www.interlog.com/~fcc/
  e-mail: fcc@interlog.com

Brainchild
Brainchild is an organization helping families with children with brain tumours. It began in 1993 with four families and today consists of 120 families. Brainchild is a volunteer organization providing support, education, and research funding. Its goals are to assist patients and their families; to inform the community about the needs of children with brain tumours as well as educate about early detection; and to seek and provide research funding to study the causes, treatments, and cures of brain tumours. Brainchild operates under the auspices of the Hospital for Sick Children.

Department of Neurosurgery
Brainchild
The Hospital for Sick Children telephone: (416) 813-7974
555 University Ave.
Toronto, Ontario M5G 1X8

S.O.L.A.C.E.
Supporting Others through Loss and Anticipatory Grief with Compassion and Empathy is a support group that comes under the umbrella of Brainchild. To date the group operates as a telephone support, meeting informally on occasion. It holds events and supports families during their time in the hospital. Presently it is organizing a newsletter. Contact may be made through Brainchild (see above).

Project Smile

Project Smile is run by a couple—Maureen and Mark Tresnak—who make and distribute quilts and toys to children with cancer while they are undergoing treatment. Their objectives are to provide security and comfort to the children; to let families know they are not alone; to provide emotional support; and to promote public awareness that children with cancer and their families need support. Project Smile deals with six oncology centres across Ontario, attempting to personalize each quilt as much as possible. The Tresnaks do much of the work themselves, with some financial and product donations from individuals and corporations. They have provided 261 children with quilts since they began in 1995. Currently, quilting guilds across the province are beginning to make and donate quilts to Project Smile.

Project Smile
1184 McIntyre St. W.
North Bay, Ontario P1B 3A8

telephone: (705) 840-5484
fax: (705) 840-5621
e-mail: psmile@efni.com
Homepage: www.efni.com/~psmile/

Centre for Health Information and Promotion (CHIP)

CHIP is located at the Hospital for Sick Children. It houses a collection of materials for families, including videos, pamphlets, books for children and adults, and manuals for school re-entry. The section devoted to families with children with cancer has been established for three years. The centre maintains close ties to support groups, the Canadian Cancer Society, and Candlelighters to ensure updated resources are current with all parties.

Centre for Health Information and Promotion
The Hospital for Sick Children
555 University Ave.
Toronto, Ontario M5G 1X8

telephone: (416) 813-6528
fax: (416) 813-6715

Web site: http://www.sickkids.on.ca/HSCWeb/CHIP/CHIPProHome.html

The Jennifer Ashleigh Foundation

The Jennifer Ashleigh Foundation is a national children's charity begun in 1990 by Norman Clements after his granddaughter, Jennifer, died at six months old of spinal muscular atrophy. The organization helps chronically and seriously ill children up to age 21 and their families with financial assistance, medical expenses, and special treatment needs.

Jennifer Ashleigh Foundation
R.R.#1 Uxbridge, Ontario L9P 1R1

telephone: (905) 640-5758 ext. 341
fax: (905) 852-4324

Starlight Children's Foundation

Starlight Foundation is an international organization with two offices in Canada. The group has been established in Canada since 1989. Starlight grants wishes to children who are chronically, critically, or seriously ill. It has also installed fun centres in pediatric wards in hospitals throughout the country. Fun centres consist of a TV, a VCR, and a Nintendo-64 unit. Starlight also provides and/or upgrades playrooms in pediatric wards in hospitals. Community Activities Network is a Starlight program of scheduled events that bring together all wish children and their families. Wishes are granted for children aged 4-18 years. Starlight relies on corporate and individual sponsors.

Starlight Children's Foundation
250 Consumer Rd. Suite 206
Toronto, Ontario M2J 4V6

telephone: (416)502-WISH
1-800-880-1004
fax: (416)502-9477
e-mail: Starlightcanada@compuserve.com

Alladin Children's Charity

Aladdin Children's Charity is a national organization established in 1995. Its goal is to grant wishes to children with terminal illnesses or life-threatening medical conditions that create the possibility the child will not survive beyond the age of 18. This organization likes to stay away from high-profile wishes, instead focusing on hospital gifts, books, small personal gifts like CD players for children who are shut in. It will also sponsor children to go to camps that meet their needs.

Aladdin Children's Charity
telephone: (416) 690-8529
fax: (416) 690-1499

The Golden Griddle Children's Charity

The primary goal is to grant wishes for terminally ill and severely disabled children aged 3-18 in Ontario. Nomination forms must be filled out, at which point the information is sent to the Golden Griddle in the child's city. Fundraising is then done at the local level featuring events such as pancake-eating contests. This program was established in 1993.

The Golden Griddle Children's Charity
505 Consumers Rd. Suite 1000
North York, Ontario M2J 4V8

telephone: (416) 493-3800 ext. 242
fax: (416) 493-3889

The Sunshine Foundation

The Sunshine Foundation grants dreams for children aged 3-19 who have a life-threatening illness or a physical disability. It was established in 1987 and serves children across Canada. It grants individual dreams, such as puppies and trips. It also has Dream Lift, which is unique from the other wish foundations.

Dream Lift is a one-day trip to Disney World and back with accompanying volunteers. Sunshine Foundation relies on corporate sponsors like Radio Shack and individuals for funding.

The Sunshine Foundation
1710-148 Fullarton St.
London, Ontario N6A 5P3

telephone: (519) 642-0990 ext. 223
1-800-461-7935
fax:(519) 642-1201

Make-A-Wish Foundation
Make-A-Wish Foundation is the largest non-profit wish-granting organization in the world. Its purpose is to fulfil special wishes of children between the ages of 2½ and 18 who have a life-threatening illness. Make-A-Wish encourages the entire family to be part of the wish experience, since parents and siblings need magical moments as much as the wish child. The foundation has established a donor program called Adopt-A-Wish, where individuals, groups, or corporations can designate their funds for a specific wish and receive non-identifying information about the child.

Make-A-Wish Foundation (SWO)
4096 Meadowbrook Dr. Unit 112
London, Ontario N6L 1G4

telephone: (519) 652-9500
fax: (519) 652-9595
e-mail: wishbone@maw.org

A Child's Voice
A Child's Voice is a non-profit organization whose goals are to support and enhance the well-being of children across Canada who are less fortunate. Children may be critically, chronically, and/or terminally ill. A Child's Voice also lends support to other groups with a similar mandate.

A Child's Voice
112 Merton St. 3rd floor
Toronto, Ontario M5S 2Z8

telephone: (416) 481-4559
1-800-837-3354

Cancer Info Service of Canadian Cancer Society
1-800-263-6750

Interpreter Services and Multicultural Resources
The Hospital for Sick Children
Toronto
telephone: (416) 813-6618

Canteen Australia Ltd
Canteen Australia is an organization especially for teens with cancer. This group has a newsletter, the *Canteen Newsletter.*

Canteen Australia
P.O. Box 83
Parkville St. Vic 3052
Australia

Canteen Newsletter
P.O. Box 1000
St Pauls NSW 2031
telephone: (02) 399-4604

Camps for Children with Cancer

Trillium Childhood Cancer Support Centre
Camp Trillium is a provincial organization with two camping sites in Ontario. It is a member of the Ontario Camping Association and the Children's Oncology Camps of America. Camp Trillium began in 1984 with a grant from the Odd Fellows and Rebekahs of Ontario and was the first of its kind offering siblings and family camps as well as summer and winter camping. It is funded by the Canadian Cancer Society and by donations from service groups. Trillium presently offers services to 1,000 participants annually, offering a range of camping programs for different ages of children and teens as well as family programs. Its mandate is to promote recreational experiences for children with cancer and their families, providing an environment that normalizes relationships, helping families in their healing, and enhancing their quality of life. There is no fee to attend the camp; however, donations are appreciated.

Camp Trillium
179 Sydenham St. Suite 2
Kingston, Ontario K7K 3M1

telephone: (613) 542-1113
fax: (613) 542-2499

Camp Oochigeas
Camp Oochigeas is an affiliate of The Hospital for Sick Children, established in 1984 as the first residential cancer camp in Canada. The camp is located at Rosseau Lake near Parry Sound, Ontario, and is for those on and off treatment. The Hospital for Sick Children has a pediatric oncologist and two oncology nurses on site at all times to administer treatment and handle emergencies. The camp also operates with a team of 145 counselling volunteers. Camp Oochigeas receives no government funding and relies on support from individuals and corporations. Campers do not pay any fee to attend the camp.

Camp Oochigeas
60 St. Clair Ave. E. Suite 404
Toronto, Ontario M4T 1N5

telephone: (416) 961-6624
(888) GO-4-OOCH
fax: (416) 961-2267
e-mail: ooch@compuserve.com

Camp Quality
Camp Quality is an international organization that began in Australia. It now has two camps in Ontario and has been operating in the province since 1987. Camp Quality is a non-profit organization that relies on fund-raising and corporate sponsorship. It is a volunteer organization offering camping experiences and year-round support for children and their families. There is no cost to campers or their families.

Camp Quality Southern Ontario
353 Forest Hill Dr. telephone: 1-800-770-5261
Kitchener, Ontario N2M 4H3

Corporate Sponsors

Amgen
Amgen is a new company, just seven years old, which is actively involved with Candlelighters Canada, supporting its biannual meetings. It has been involved in patient education work with Candlelighters and provides colouring books and videos for children with cancer. It contributed financial support to the Children with Cancer Conference held in Montreal in July-August 1998.

Amgen
6733 Mississauga Rd. Suite 303 telephone: (905) 542-7277
Mississauga, Ontario L5N 6J5

Glaxo Wellcomes
Glaxo Wellcomes works with both the Canadian Cancer Society and Candlelighters to channel funding for children with cancer. It has established a foundation to provide funding chiefly for hospice and palliative care.

Glaxo Wellcomes
7333 Mississauga Rd. N. telephone: (905) 819-3000
Mississauga, Ontario L5N 6L4

Medsep
Medsep manufactures blood bags and has sponsored workshops with the Hemophiliac Society and Candlelighters to encourage awareness for patients and parents regarding blood transfusions and alternatives.

Medsep
1785 Altavista Dr. Suite 101 telephone: 1-800-465-8555
Ottawa, Ontario K1G 3Y6

Astra

Astra is a pharmaceutical company that donates funds to various events that promote awareness of childhood cancer. It has been a sponsor of Candlelighters and was also a sponsor at the Montreal conference on childhood cancer in July 1998.

Astra
1004 Middlegate Rd. telephone: (905) 566-4015
Mississauga, Ontario L4Y 1M4

Pizza Hut

Pizza Hut corporate restaurants is the sole corporate sponsor for Candlelighters. This relationship was established in June 1997 and the relationship is in the building stage. Pizza Hut supported Candlelighters Walk in 1997 and the two groups are planning further events. Pizza Hut encourages promotions at the local level for a community focus.

Pizza Hut
telephone: (416) 674-0367